D1020531

Benchmarks of Fairness
for Health Care Reform

Benchmarks of Fairness for Health Care Reform

NORMAN DANIELS
DONALD W. LIGHT
RONALD L. CAPLAN

New York   Oxford
OXFORD UNIVERSITY PRESS
1996

Oxford University Press

Oxford   New York
Athens   Auckland   Bangkok   Bombay
Calcutta   Cape Town   Dar es Salaam   Delhi
Florence   Hong Kong   Istanbul   Karachi
Kuala Lumpur   Madras   Madrid   Melbourne
Mexico City   Nairobi   Paris   Singapore
Taipei   Tokyo   Toronto

and associated companies in
Berlin   Ibadan

Copyright © 1996 by Oxford University Press, Inc.

Published by Oxford University Press, Inc.,
198 Madison Avenue, New York, New York 10016

Oxford is a registered trademark of Oxford University Press

Library of Congress Cataloging-in-Publication Data
Daniels, Norman, 1942–
Benchmarks of fairness for health care reform / Norman Daniels,
Donald W. Light, Ronald L. Caplan.
p.   cm. Includes bibliographical references and index.
ISBN 0-19-510237-1
1. Health planning—Moral and ethical aspects.
2. Health care reform—Moral and ethical aspects.
I. Light, Donald, 1942–
II. Caplan, Ronald L.
III. Title.
RA394.9.D36   1996
362.1—dc20   95-47820

9 8 7 6 5 4 3 2 1

Printed in the United States of America
on acid-free paper

Preface

This book is the product of collaboration by a philosopher, a sociologist, and an economist. It could not have been written by any one of us. Just as we could not have written it without each other, we could not have done so without the help of others, both institutions and individuals.

The project had its genesis with a prescient suggestion by Donald Light late in 1991, before health care reform had emerged at center stage on the national agenda, that Norman Daniels collaborate with him to develop a scorable way to assess the fairness of health care reform proposals. This suggestion lead to support from the Robert Wood Johnson Foundation (Grant 20578) during 1993 to 1994 for the research and the writing of the report on which this book is based. We owe them our greatest collective debt.

Each of us has further debts to acknowledge.

Norman Daniels

In January 1993, while on a Tufts Sabbatical leave, with support as a Fellow in the Program in Ethics and the Professions at Harvard University, I wrote "Justice and the Assessment of National Health Insurance Proposals," which was delivered at a conference at Harvard Medical School in March 1993. I wish to thank both Tufts University and Harvard University for their support. During March and April of 1993, the "design principles" developed in that paper were discussed by the Ethics Working Group of the Clinton Administration Health Care Task Force, of which I was a member. Building on that paper and their own diverse experience, members of that group developed a set of principles that should govern the Clinton proposal and reform more generally. The results of that work were published by the White House Domestic Policy Council (1993:11) as the "Ethical Foundations of Health Reform." A more careful presentation of those principles can be found in Brock and Daniels (1994), and I wish to offer particular thanks to Dan Brock and other members of the Ethics Working Group. A revision of the original Harvard conference paper can be found in Daniels (1995, chapter 8).

During the summer and fall of 1993, Don Light and I modified and refined these early lists of principles into the benchmarks discussed in this book. During 1994, with additional help from Ron Caplan, we refined the benchmarks, developed criteria for scoring them, and attempted an initial analysis of several health reform proposals. These formed the basis of our report for the Robert Wood Johnson Foundation (Daniels, Light, and Caplan 1994). After the failure of reform in 1994, Ron Caplan undertook the study of current trends that forms the basis of chapter 6. We also wish to thank Jackie Caplan and Typagraphics for assistance in preparation of figures and tables.

Donald Light

The seed of this book was planted in 1986 to 1988 when I witnessed systematic efforts to dismantle one of the nation's oldest and largest community-rated insurance pools. These included premium increases that discriminated against women and older policy holders. As the Commissioner of Insurance approved the increases, I set about organizing through the New Jersey Public Health Association a subscriber's protest that in time included the AARP, the NAACP, NOW, and the New Jersey Council of Churches. In defining the issues for the public against state officials who said the increases were "fair," I realized that both I and others needed to know a good deal more about the issues of distributive justice. I am therefore grateful to Donald Daniels, Kenneth Merin, Thomas Kean and the New Jersey Public Health Association, especially Sylvia Herz and John Carlano, for launching this sociologist of comparative health care systems into the field of distributive justice. Half of my royalties will go to the association in appreciation of their unflagging support. At a more personal, deeper level, I am indebted to my family for tolerating my immersion into this seven-year project.

A fellowship at Oxford gave me the chance to read moral philosophy, and a successful legal challenge that forced the restoration of community rates for several hundred thousand individual subscribers seemed to vindicate two years' efforts. A retaliatory effort the next year to raise the community rates by four times the increases in medical expenditures provided an opportunity to address new forms of distributive justice, and a second citizens' campaign got the increases rolled back to one-quarter their original amount. Eventually, the legislature recreated the entire original community-rated pool in modern guise.

With the encouragement of Professor Robert Socolow at Princeton University, I applied for and received the DeCamp Fellowship in Ethics and the Life Sciences. This provided me with an opportunity to participate in the circle of moral philosophy at the Princeton's Rockefeller Center for Human Values and to spawn the irreverent idea of transposing a concept of justice into benchmarks, with notches for scoring the relative fairness of health care systems or their reform. Besides Professor Socolow's invaluable support and advice, my chairman, William F. Ranieri, and my dean, Frederick O. Humphrey, at the School of Osteopathic Medicine that makes up part of the University of Medicine and Dentistry of New Jersey, provided unwavering encouragement. In trying fiscal times, this was not easy, and I am indebted to their enlightened sponsorship. In return, I am giving the other half of my royalties to my department.

Beth Stevens, senior program officer of the Robert Wood Johnson Foundation, saw promise in our atypical proposal and shepherded it through the review process. We greatly appreciate her good advice as well as the support of Joel C. Cantor, Director of Evaluation Research, and Steven A. Schroeder, president of the foundation. Finally, we wish to thank Jeffrey W. House, vice president of Oxford University Press, for seeing the potential for this book in our report to the foundation and for giving us the opportunity to realize that potential.

Ronald Caplan

I would like to thank Drew Harris and Sol Swanger for their support throughout the writing of this book. I could always count on Drew for invigorating discussion and useful references. Sol was the perfect host at our marathon meeting at his house. I am especially grateful to my family—Jackie, Joel, and Sarah—for their encouragement and love.

Contents

Benchmarks of Fairness
for Health Care Reform

1

Fairness and the Politics of Health Care Reform

Our aim in this book is to put fairness on the table as an issue in the national debate about health care reform and the design of our health care system. Specifically, we develop a tool consisting of scorable benchmarks for assessing ten dimensions of the fairness of health care reform proposals. Its purpose is not to moralize or to grab the high moral ground for hidden political purposes. Rather, it is to provide a framework that facilitates debate and understanding and clarifies what social values are at stake, often hidden, in the complex details of health policy.

In light of the failure of reform efforts in the 103rd Congress, we expect that some readers may already be saying, "Here they come, Don Quixote, Sancho Panza, and Rozinante, tilting at windmills. What health care reform proposals? What national debate? What concerns about fairness?"

Our premise is that health care reform remains a live issue in the public's mind and that greater clarity about how our social values are reflected in reform is a necessary condition for improving the system. One hypothesis we explore briefly in this chapter is that the lack of public clarity about issues of fairness made it easier for opponents of reform to derail it in the 103rd Congress. Of course, there is an alternative hypothesis—that American values cannot support a comprehensive reform that includes universal insurance coverage, that we are too individualistic or even selfish. In chapter 2 we reject that hypothesis. We believe that a core American value, a widely shared concern for equality of opportunity, provides the key to understanding what a fair health care system would look like. In chapter 3 we develop our matrix of benchmarks, clarifying the moral and empirical assumptions that underlie various judgments about the fairness of reform proposals. In chapters 4 and 5 we illustrate use of the benchmarks by assessing the types of comprehensive reform that were under consideration in the 103rd Congress. Finally, in chapter 6, we apply the benchmarks to current market-driven trends.

A Close Encounter of the National Health Insurance Kind

During the first two years of the Clinton presidency, the nation experienced a close encounter with national health insurance, an idea often thought alien to American society and culture. Not only did President Clinton develop an elaborate bill and submit it to Congress, but several major alternative proposals, representing varying degrees of reform from comprehensive to modestly incremental, were submitted from across the political spectrum to the 103rd Congress. All the political players clearly thought comprehensive reform was on the agenda, whether they supported it or saw it as a threat and fought to hold it to a minimum. The general public, including consumers and providers of health care, also had high expectations that some form of comprehensive reform would take place.

Many people seemed to understand how the twin problems of spiraling costs and lack of insurance coverage feed on one another. Rising costs make access difficult for many. To contain costs, access is restricted in both subtle and not so subtle ways. As many lose insurance coverage or have their coverage reduced through restrictions, payment caps, higher co-payments, and related techniques (Light 1992b), providers of care raise charges and shift costs to those who are better insured and can pay more. Cost shifting may save money for one institution, but it does not save money for the economy as a whole. Comprehensive reform was the only way, many came to think, to solve both problems at once.

Forces as diverse as the uninsured, employers, organized labor, state governments, and many health care providers, including many insurers, were all on the side of some form of comprehensive reform, although for very different reasons. The uninsured—largely poor working people—wanted the same benefits that better-off workers had. Many workers with insurance wanted reform because they recognize that job loss or job change threatened their assurance of coverage, especially for family members with prior health conditions. Clinton's main sales pitch was to this group of insured workers—his health security card promised portable security for all.

Large and small employers that provided health care benefits wanted the rate of cost increases constrained. They felt it was unfair that health costs of the uninsured were shifted to them. Organized labor also wanted costs constrained, since negotiating to maintain health care benefits eliminated the possibility of increasing real wages; indeed, in recent years, about 75 percent of all strikes have been about benefits. At the same time, unions feared any reform that might reduce their benefits. State governments looked to the federal government for relief from the rising costs of Medicaid, especially the rapidly rising costs of the elderly needing long-term care. Many physicians and other health care providers wished they could be rid of the huge cost and time burden of processing insurance forms and negotiating with insurers regarding clinical decisions for their patients. Hospitals saw universal coverage as a solution to the problem of providing un-reimbursed care in a context where cost-shifting had become more difficult. Some large insurers saw the chance to grow in a more competitive, larger health care market, provided the reform retained a large private insurance market.

With this convergence of forces, if not of reasons, how could reform fail? Expectations seemed justifiably high. But they had seemed so twenty years earlier, when both parties submitted major bills for universal coverage, leading many to think comprehensive reform was just around the corner (Rivlin 1974; Iglehart 1976).

Nevertheless, as in previous close encounters with this alien idea, expectations were dashed. The diverse forces supporting reform pulled apart. The uninsured formed no grass roots organization that could make their numbers felt. They hired no lobbyists and made no campaign contributions. There was also no effort to organize them or to appeal to them from above, including from the White House. Some of the uninsured, clearly moved by the scare tactics of their "small business" employers, became fearful that employer mandates might actually cost them their jobs. These employers—who included such "small" entities as the combined McDonalds franchises—fought dollar and lobbyist against any form of employer mandate. They opposed the mandate even when it was well cushioned by concessions President Clinton included in his proposal to shield the most vulnerable employers from the full burden of financing care. Large employers backed away. Even an important organization of Fortune 500 corporations, the Business Roundtable, was pushed to oppose the Clinton proposal because of the influence of some large insurers (Judis 1995).

Insurers, whom President Clinton had hoped would not attack his plan because he opted to retain a largely private insurance sector, split. Though a few large insurers, who thought they would gain from the plan, remained supportive, most insurers attacked comprehensive reform vigorously, not just through lobbying, but through the brilliant, multimillion dollar "Harry and Louise" television advertising campaign. These ads countered Clinton's claim that health reform was aimed at protecting everyone's security. They portrayed a middle-class couple speculating about how a "government run" plan would take away their choices and the quality of their care. Universal coverage was thus portrayed as a benefit for "them," the poor, but one that hurts "us," everyone else. These ads divided working people against themselves.

Many physician groups, especially those representing specialists, were fearful that comprehensive reform might work against their interests, especially if managed care arrangements were strengthened. Much antagonism to Clinton's plan was generated by physicians and other providers whose lobbyists had felt shut out of the task force that the administration had assembled to work out the details of a plan that affected one-seventh of the economy. The intention of relying on "experts" free from the lobbying efforts of vested interests was portrayed as "secretive" and perceived by many as such.

Finally, many supporters of universal coverage, including some physician groups, could not agree on a particular plan to support. Supporters of a Canadian-style single-payer plan attacked Clinton's plan for its complexity and its threat to "choice" of provider. The lack of unity by those in favor of universal coverage may have added to the growing public anxiety about "managed competition" and managed care.

The failure of the 103rd Congress to act on comprehensive reform, despite widespread public support for the idea, at least early in that Congress, must be credited to a significant extent to the explicit strategy proposed by William Kristol, the leading conservative strategist. He argued that Republicans should claim that there is no "crisis" in the health care system, should back away from comprehensive reform, and should oppose "sight unseen" compromise proposals aimed at comprehensive reform (see Starr 1995). He foresaw that the effect of failure to reform the system would be blamed on Clinton and his "big government" proposal, not on Republican "obstructionism," especially if the "obstructionism" was portrayed as necessary to "save us" from catastrophic government interference in health care. Obstruction became a virtue, not a vice, even to a public that railed against gridlock.

Responsibility for the failure of reform does not just lie with those who actively opposed it. It also lies with those who ineffectively supported it and underestimated the force of the attacks on it. Neither Clinton nor the proponents of comprehensive reform in Congress, in both parties, made a serious effort to save the coalition of forces favoring comprehensive reform. Despite the appeal of Clinton's national speeches for his proposal, no sustained campaign to reach the public and explain his complex proposal was launched, and the field was largely left to the television campaign of insurers. This was clearly a context in which strong presidential leadership was needed. Clinton had to appeal directly and actively to a public supportive of the general idea of reform.

Such a campaign would have required much more than the occasional "big" national speech. Perhaps it was impossible for a president as beleaguered as Clinton to launch that campaign; or perhaps it was a failure of leadership not to try. Nor was Clinton adept at a seeking a compromise with moderates early enough to undercut Kristol's strategy, before it lured away or undermined those moderates who favored some version of comprehensive reform. (This point is easy to suggest in hindsight; at the time, had Clinton abandoned universal coverage or other key features of his plan, he would have lost many of his supporters.) Kristol's brilliant and cynical strategy worked, despite the fact that many scoffed at it when it was first announced. Clinton's failure to produce health care "security for all" played a significant role in his party's loss of both houses of Congress later that year.

In the wake of attacks on Clinton's plan, exit polls of voters who elected the 104th Congress revealed a confused public. Though the public had not abandoned its desire for reform, even comprehensive reform, it was much more fearful than a year earlier that comprehensive reform of the sort proposed by the president might reduce the quality of its health care. It also seemed clear that the public was confused by the complexity of reform itself. The public had not seen how to connect is concerns and its values with a specific type of reform proposal.

A Question of Values

Is the American public unable to support reform because of its values? Is it "too individualistic," too selfish and lacking in social solidarity to support a universal coverage scheme? Does it have "insufficient empathy" (Roberts 1993:156)? Answering "yes" to these questions provides an ungenerous, but often made, interpretation of our social values and the cause of the failure of reform.

Or was the American public confused by claims exaggerating harms to the system and to benefits already enjoyed by many? This was probably the most lobbied against and advertised against legislative reform in our history. Could an American public clearer about the details of reform and the way in which reform reflected its values support a national health care insurance plan? Answering "yes" to these questions is the basis for a generous interpretation of the public frame of mind.

But which interpretation is true?

That is a hard question. None of the authors of this book is confident that we know which interpretation of the public mood is true. None has the expertise or hubris to attempt a definitive analysis of the reasons reform failed or to assign blame for the failure. Like others, however, we have our opinions and have not been shy about noting some of them. We return to the question again in the next chapter.

Our hypothesis is that it is particularly difficult to decide between these alternative interpretations, since clear discussion of the values underlying reform, especially the values of justice and fairness, was never on the public agenda and never a central part of the policy debate in Congress. As a result, the effect on our values—the "cost" in values—of reform or of failure to reform was not clear to the public. We believe that a better outcome in health care reform requires the public to have a clearer picture of the values underlying different aspects of reform. This would not have guaranteed a successful reform in the 103rd Congress, nor will it guarantee such success in the future. Still, without that moral clarity, failure is likely. Greater clarity about fairness would, however, have changed the character of the national debate. If we are right, we might now be writing about how to implement particular reforms, or about how to measure their effects on the fairness of the system, rather than about the prospects for any reform.

In any case, our project in this book is primarily forward-, not backward-looking. Our most recent close encounter with national health insurance will probably not be our last, despite the hostile climate to such reform in the 104th Congress. Many of the fundamental problems that underlay earlier claims about a health care "crisis" and a need for comprehensive reform remain, despite, and to some extent even because of, the extensive market-driven reorganization that is underway. Despite a growing economy, nearly two million more Americans have lost insurance coverage since the reform effort began in 1993 (Freudenheim 1995b; Hellander et. al. 1995; Bradsher 1995). There is increasing evidence that lack of insurance coverage has a negative effect on health outcomes for the uninsured patients, despite the fact that many uninsured secure some form of needed care (Hadley, Steinberg, and Feder 1991; Franks, Clancy, and Gold 1993; Stoddard, Peter, and Newacheck 1994). There is conflicting evidence and opinion about the degree to which health care cost increases have slowed or merely been shifted and about the degree to which these are short- or long-term effects. The market-driven reorganization is perceived as a threat by many physicians and hospitals. Many patients—who believed the "Harry and Louise" ads sponsored by insurers, and thought that only "government run" reform would push them into managed care arrangements—are now finding that the loss of choice and quality that Harry and Louise prophesied has come true for them but without any of the benefits government reform promised. Many people are finding they are losing important "choices." They are finding it more difficult to secure important benefits, such as needed mental health care services, through their new insurance and provider arrangements.

Putting Fairness on the Table

Our project in this book is forward-looking in this sense: we develop a tool for examining the fairness of health care reform proposals. Our premise is that this tool would help those struggling to understand competing reform proposals to see what important values, aspects of fairness in particular, are at stake. Greater clarity about this crucial issue would help everyone see better what we are committed to when we think about reforming as complex an institution as the health care system. Greater clarity and clearer commitments on issues of value or principle might not have saved some version of reform in the last attempt, but we believe they would have helped. We believe that future attempts at reform will also benefit from better ways of evaluating competing approaches.

In that spirit, we propose this tool—ten "benchmarks" of fairness—that can be used to score reform proposals (see chapters 4 and 5) or assess various trends in our unreformed and market-driven system (see chapter 6). This report card gives a glimpse of performance on several dimensions of the complex idea of fairness in a system. The tool is not perfect, by any means. It would gain considerably from discussion, revision, and improvement— which we hope this book will stimulate. We also think the tool, appropriately modified, has other uses as well, for example, helping us to make comparisons among types of health care systems.

We aim to put fairness on the table alongside other criteria for weighing the merits of a given health care reform. The benchmarks we propose organize many of the values emphasized by others (cf. Priester 1992; Marmor 1994) into a single, coherent framework with a scoring procedure so that for the first time core values for reform get translated into a comparative score for alternative reform proposals. The reform proposals presented in the 103rd Congress, and the ones we are likely to encounter in the future, range from "large government" approaches to attempts to manage private insurance markets on a large scale to modest "gap filling" proposals. They are usually debated largely in terms of what will work best for raising money, containing costs, and improving health outcomes, or with reference to what political concessions must be made to the big players, such as the health insurance industry. Now they can be debated in terms of their fairness as well.

Concerns about fairness are often implicit—and sometimes hidden—in many features of competing proposals and debates about them. For example, many objected to an employer mandate because of the burdens it would impose on small businesses. They complained that the extra cost of providing coverage would cost jobs to the workers for whom insurance was sought, either because of a lack of job growth or even because of bankruptcy. On the other side, larger employers complained about the shifting of costs to them: uninsured workers still received medical care and the cost of that care was covered in part by raising charges to employees with insurance coverage.

Sometimes the term "fairness" would surface in this exchange. Opponents of a mandate argued that it is unfair to require them to accept burdens that threatened their business. Proponents argued that shifting costs to them was unfair, that fairness required all to pay their share. But in the public arena, no meaningful discussion of the fundamental issues of fairness involved in employer mandates ever took place.

In a similar fashion, issues of fairness were hidden in discussions of the appropriate benefit package to be included in health care reform. Proposals that had comprehensive, uniform benefit packages were attacked for being expensive or because they involved government regulation that "burdened" some people with more coverage than they wanted and that tied the hands of insurers seeking more efficient delivery. Proponents replied that most people wanted these benefits and that the costs were manageable and had to be covered since they would be paid somewhere in the system by someone.

The terminology of this debate about the benefit package is primarily the language of economic analysis: costs, demand, competition, regulation. Only occasionally would we hear that it was unfair to restrict market choices in this way, or, from the other side, that it was unfair, unjust or inequitable not to include needed mental health or long-term care services. No serious and clear debate about what justice or fairness involved took place.

Financing is another area in which issues of fairness are central but rarely discussed. Many people view medical insurance as simply a way of buying security: a given package of security should cost one family what it costs another, just like a refrigerator, a computer, or a car. Seen in this way, premiums are an appropriate way to distribute the costs of medical insurance. If we want to give everyone access to insurance, we may have to subsidize premiums for low-income people, but beyond that, it costs what it costs. Others think we have social obligations to assure people access to health care, whether or not they can pay for it and regardless of their levels of risk. They believe that this social obligation should be financed in a way that reflects people's ability to pay. Specifically, we should find as progressively financed a tax base as we can. But the issue of financing was never discussed as an issue of fairness in the distribution of benefits and burdens.

Instead, it was cast in terms of "more taxes" and "big government" versus less of both.

Fairness is submerged in the deliberations about health care reform for three main reasons. First, in the political arena, we expect people to pursue their interests. We think that if people do not protect themselves and their interests, no one else will. We might hope that in an ideal world people would be publicly spirited, but this is the real world. As realists, we do not expect such behavior. We still hope that the public good emerges when the political process reconciles our individual and group pursuits of our separate interests. As realists, we also know that our elected representatives will ally themselves with particular groups and interests. This is constituency politics, the politics of interests. Money talks. Ideally, but only ideally, we hope that our representatives can adopt a more detached or neutral societal perspective, surveying and pursuing the public good. We simply cross our fingers and hope that the public good emerges from the process.

Of course, we expect individuals, groups, and politicians to pursue interests in a way that is constrained by certain basic considerations of justice. We expect that there will remain a respect for basic liberties, due process, and equality of opportunity. We erect constitutional and institutional protections to provide these constraints. Still, we expect the pursuit of individual and group interests. We listen to people when they complain some policy or reform is unfair. But we are somewhat skeptical, even cynical. We expect counterclaims about fairness from competing parties, but we devalue and discount them almost automatically. We expect the coinage of fairness itself to be debased by self-serving interpretations of principle.

A careful debate about fairness requires deliberation and some detachment from personal interests. Ideally, public discussion would provide a forum, both in the media and in the legislature, for such a careful deliberation and judicious detachment. It would encourage adopting a societal perspective. But the power of media, especially the electronic media, to reduce debate to soundbites, and the power of lobbyists to undermine the kind of detachment and pursuit of the public good that we would like to see in our representatives, and the very complexity of an issue so vast as health care reform—all these factors combine to hide from us real concerns about social justice and fairness.

A second reason that fairness is submerged in the debate about health care is that mainstream economics, divorced from its origins in political philosophy, particularly in the United States, lacks the necessary concepts and vocabulary for such a discourse. According to neoclassical economics, all values, including justice and fairness, lie outside the market (Glaser 1993). Consequently, they get converted into "political" decisions about income distribution. The focus of economic analysis is on assuring efficiency and tampering with imperfect markets to improve it. While efficiency can contribute to the fairness of a system, efficient systems are not necessarily fair.

A related way in which economics buries consideration of value, including fairness, is by construing all choices as expressions of "preference" or "taste." In the extreme, the Nobel-prize-winning economist, Milton Friedman (1962:110–113), compared a taste for opera or the blues with a taste for hiring blacks or whites. If public taste works against the market value of blacks, he argued, they have no more reason to complain than opera singers have to complain that more people like blues than opera. Similarly, it is presumably no more than a "preference" for not letting people die in the streets that leads us to treat the uninsured with money collected from the insured. This prevailing brand of economics has little room for moral vocabulary or a hierarchy of moral values. It also has no way to consider criteria, including those of fairness, that are not part of prevailing tastes and preferences.

The economists' vision has captured the domain of policy discussion. It purports to cover the whole field of the facts of the matter. It claims to tell us everything that is relevant about how things work and what is real. Anything outside this economic domain is portrayed as unscientific. Values lie in this outside domain. Our dominant paradigm of policy analysis thus squeezes any rigorous discussion of values out of careful consideration.

The third major reason that fairness is submerged in the current debates is that people confuse fairness with "fair deals." There is an inclination to think that the process of political "dealing," of arriving at compromises reflecting the competing interests of the big players in the health care field, is a way of arriving at a fair outcome, that is, one to which all the big players can agree. This confusion is fed, in obvious ways, by what we cited as the first reason, our expectation that the political arena is intended as a domain for the pursuit of separate interests.

But fairness is not whatever emerges from these deals. There are deeper issues of fairness, reflected in notions like a "right to health care" or meeting the range of health care needs people have, and these concerns about fairness should act as constraints on the acceptable outcomes of making political deals. Confusing "fair deals" with fairness reflects our cynicism: politics is not ethics; it is power. Politics may displace ethics, but it cannot replace it. It is crucial when addressing fundamental issues of the structure of our society that we insist that justice regulate politics. That is our intention here, to provide a tool for thinking through the implications of justice and fairness (we use the terms interchangeably) in the design of the health care system.

Our goal in this book is to include fairness in the debate about health care. To do that, we need to explain what fairness requires in the design of a health care system. We may then develop measures of fairness that can be used in a practical way to assess alternate proposals for health care reform. In the next chapter, we argue that a central theme about fairness in American culture and law is to assure people fair access to opportunities in life. Our avowed social obligation to guarantee equality of opportunity actually provides the basis for assuring fairness in the design of health care systems. A system aimed at protecting equality of opportunity will aim at keeping people functioning as close to normal as possible, but within the context of reasonable resource constraints.

This view has important implications for the distribution of health care benefits and the burdens of financing them. We recast these implications as a series of "benchmarks of fairness." By specifying criteria for measuring how reform proposals satisfy these benchmarks, we provide a matrix for assessing the fairness of alternative health care reform proposals along ten important dimensions of fairness. This matrix can be used for other purposes than assessing the fairness of alternative health care proposals. For example, with some modifications of the criteria and the scale, it might be used to compare systems in different countries.

Our central purpose in this book, however, is to show the value of this tool for thinking about health care reform (or its absence) in the United States. After explaining these benchmarks, we use them to score four of the proposals that had been before Congress in the 103rd Congress. These specific proposals are clearly dead, but they represent an array of types of reform proposals. By examining them in detail, we illustrate the power of the matrix to examine matters of fairness. We also put the matrix to a slightly different use in chapter 6, where we assess current trends in the U.S. system after the failure of national reform.

2

American Values and the Fairness of Health Care Reform

Are Americans Indifferent to Fairness?

Are Americans concerned enough about fairness and social justice to assess health care reform in terms of those values?

The United States remains the only advanced industrial country in the world that fails to assure universal access to medical services. In the past, this fact has prompted some commentators to suggest that Americans lack the culture—the values—to support such a system, or at least to charge that our values must be an important part of the explanation of the absence of universal coverage (see Feldstein 1994:254; Rothman 1993). They claim that we are more "individualistic" than other countries and lack the social solidarity that leads people to share the burdens and benefits of such a system (cf. Evans 1993). We are so intent on protecting our rights as individuals to pursue "life, liberty and happiness" free from interference by others or our government that we are unwilling to support each other even with regard to fundamental needs.

This charge about American culture has resurfaced in the wake of the failure of the 103rd Congress to enact a comprehensive reform (cf. Brown 1994; Reinhardt 1995a), and it is buttressed by the wave of spending reductions in social services approved by the 104th Congress. The "ungenerous" interpretation of the public mood after the 1994 election, noted in the previous chapter, fits with this view. Of course, no one ascribes sole responsibility, and perhaps not even primary responsibility, to our values alone (see the sophisticated accounts in Blendon, Brodie, and Benson 1995 and in Schlesinger and Lee 1993), but an ungenerous view of our values is a common feature of accounts of the reform failure. Is it true that we just do

15

not have the values it takes to create what other countries see as a decent and fair system of social support?

If this accusation is true, then our project in this book loses its practical purpose. We intend our benchmarks to help everyone better understand what issues of justice and fairness underlie the complex elements of health care reform. The "individualistic" public portrayed in the ungenerous accusation would have little interest in our project or the tool we develop. To clear some ground for our effort, we must briefly address the ungenerous view of American culture.

This pessimistic picture cannot simply be dismissed. Many other advanced, industrialized countries have much more robust "safety nets" for their poorest and sickest members than we have. Their institutions seem to suggest a greater sense of community, a greater sense of social solidarity (not to be confused with nationalism) than ours (Evans 1993). This contrast, however, is not the whole story. For one thing, there is a chicken-and-egg problem: Does culture create institutions, or do institutions foster culture? The answer is "both." Broadly held attitudes that the government can effectively promote social welfare and that everyone must be concerned with the welfare of others make it easier to establish social welfare institutions, but good experiences with such institutions also strengthen attitudes that support them. More to the point, facts about public attitudes and values in the United States may not be the most important part of an explanation of the failure to reform our health care system in particular. Facts about particular interest groups and their wealth and power may be more important.

The ungenerous claims about American culture ignore important facts about our society and its institutions that point us toward another conclusion. In poll after poll, over many years, an overwhelming majority of Americans say they believe no one should be denied needed medical services because of an inability to pay. Even in the polls following the 1994 election, a strong majority avows the commitment to health care as a right, and other views consistent with substantial reform, even when they backed away from specific reform proposals (see Blendon, Brodie, and Benson 1995).

"It is just lip service," supporters of the ungenerous view of American values are quick to reply. "If these really are American values and commitments, where are the institutions to back them up? Why don't we have universal coverage within a national health insurance system?" These critics insist that we we put our money where we say our values lie.

In fact, we have "put up" some institutions—Medicaid and Medicare—that reflect, at least palely, the more generous values we avow in the polls. Medicaid provides a means-tested system of medical insurance for the very poorest members of society. For thirty years, this "entitlement" program has recognized the right of every Medicaid eligible person to medical services covered by the program. This partial recognition has clearly inadequate in many ways. It leaves many who are poor by federal definitions, as well as the working poor, ineligible for coverage. It leaves Medicaid underfunded, reducing real access to services for those who are covered and threatening their quality of care. For example, reimbursement rates to physicians are so low that many simply refuse to treat Medicaid patients at all. Still, Medicaid is more than just talk; it is money, a lot of money. In fact, rapidly rising state Medicaid budgets, largely driven by the long-term care costs of the eligible elderly, have been one reason states looked to comprehensive national reform for budget relief.

Medicare, too, puts money where we say our values lie. It is a universal, public insurance system that covers our elderly population for acute medical needs without regard to ability to pay (although it requires substantial out-of-pocket payments). An entitlement program, Medicare recognizes the right of all eligible Americans over age sixty-five to have their medical needs met, and it requires the whole working population to support that entitlement through a payroll tax.

Medicare, despite flaws, is a program that senior Americans fight vigorously to protect and that other Americans are reluctant to threaten, despite its rapidly rising costs and the burdens they impose on the working population. Unlike Medicaid, it is an all-class program: rich and poor alike among the elderly share in its benefits. This fact helps explain why Medicare has until now fared better than Medicaid during periods in which social service budgets have been cut. In fact, Medicare is a model of the type of comprehensive reform we failed to achieve in the 103rd Congress: a tax-based scheme that recognizes the idea that health care is a fundamental good that all are entitled to receive.

The existence of Medicare and Medicaid show that Americans are not so uncommitted to social justice or fairness or support of others in need as the ungenerous view suggests. Although we fall well short of living up to the values we claim to have, the ungenerous attack on American values overreaches and oversimplifies. It fails to explain our support for Medicare and Medicaid, but more than that, it fails to explain why the majority of working people do not act in their own interest by improving their own security and extending universal coverage to each other. We should seek better explanations for why we do not have a universal national health insurance scheme, after several close encounters, than merely blaming people for being too selfish and claiming that universal coverage is alien and un-American.

Better explanations for the failure of national health care lie in the fact that comprehensive reform threatens powerful, wealthy interests. As we noted in the first chapter, health care reform threatened many insurers and many special interests among health care providers. It threatened small business. Opposing reform provided an opportunity for conservatives, both Republicans and Democrats, to strengthen their hand in Congress. We believe the better explanations for the failure of this reform, as for previous attempts, lie, at least to a significant degree, in the willingness of those who profit from the existing system to fight effectively for its preservation against the common good (see Judis 1995; Blendon, Brodie, and Benson 1995; Starr 1995). Others already have provided such accounts for past close encounters with national health insurance (Starr 1982), and the full story of our most recent failure has yet to be told in detail. Our task here, however, is not to provide those explanations in detail but to simply suggest they exist and to oppose hasty, uncritical acceptance of the pessimistic view of American values.

If Americans give more than lip service to the kinds of values that underlie comprehensive reform, including universal coverage, then a careful discussion of how issues of fairness are at stake in health care reform will make it harder to confuse the public and deflect attention from needed reforms. The discussion, and the tool we provide, will help arm the public against those whose interests make them determined to foil reform at all costs. There is both room and need for an analytic tool to assess the fairness of health care reform.

Equal Opportunity: A Key American Value

We believe that American values not only leave clear ground for our project but actually provide a deep and secure foundation for concerns about fairness in health care reform. Our starting point among those values, however, is not the avowed belief of many Americans that health care is a "right and not a privilege." We view that belief as the conclusion, not the starting point, of a discussion about what we owe each other by way of fair treatment in our health care system. Instead, we seek a foundation for the claim that health care is a right. The deeper beliefs and values that support such a right will also help us answer important questions about it. What are its scope and limits? When should we take money from some people to cover the health care needs of others? When is it not appropriate or required? Does a medical need give rise to unlimited claims on the resources of others?

Our commitment to equality of opportunity, a widely avowed and institutionalized feature of our system of public values, provides an answer to these questions about the limits of our obligations, as well as a solid foundation for the belief that health care is a right (see Daniels 1985).

This is our central claim in this chapter. We do not simply mean that *if* we are obliged to meet health care needs, then we are obliged to do so in a nondiscriminatory way that reflects our commitment to equality of opportunity. Such a weak appeal to equality of opportunity does not imply that we are in any way obliged to meet everyone's health care needs or that there is a right to health care. Rather, our stronger claim is that we are obliged to meet health care needs because doing so is an important way of protecting our opportunities, and we are obliged to protect equality of opportunity. Equality of opportunity thus provides a deep foundation for a social obligation to meet health care needs. Before arguing for our claim, we want to emphasize that this foundation is quintessentially American in its flavor.

At the heart of our social concerns about fairness, including much legislation we enacted in the middle of this century, is the idea that we must create a "level playing field" free from obstacles based on "irrelevant" facts about individuals, such as race, gender, religion, age, or disabilities. On such a field, if people have the requisite talents, skills, and determination, they have a fair chance to succeed. This view of equality of opportunity is essentially *procedural*. It says that an outcome is fair or just if the process or procedure that produced it is fair. The view is used to justify a system in which unequal outcomes—even very unequal outcomes—are considered morally acceptable. It is morally acceptable that there are winners and losers, even in races where the prize is a share of fundamental social goods, provided the race is fair to all participants. For example, since major rewards in our society derive from the jobs and offices we hold, the competition for securing these positions must be fair. Specifically, "irrelevant" features of individuals—gender, race, and so on—must be ignored, and capabilities relevant to the positions sought should determine selection.

Over the past forty years, the Constitution and legislation have been used to make this value central to our thinking about fairness—in housing, education, hiring and firing, and voting. At least in their laws, even if not always in their practice, most Americans support the view that individual traits like race, sex, age, or disability should not be allowed to lessen opportunities in life.

In thinking about this issue, we need to distinguish between two notions of equality of opportunity (see Rawls 1971 for further discussion of these distinctions). We protect *formal* equality of opportunity when we insist that race, gender, age, or disabilities should not play a role in determining our opportunities. Formal equality of opportunity imposes only a negative obligation. We must refrain from allowing gender, race, and other traits to interfere with the direct assessment of relevant capabilities. In contrast, *fair* equality of opportunity involves a positive obligation to eliminate residual unfairness in the distribution of capabilities. We assure each other fair equality of opportunity when we offer assistance wherever unfair practices regarding race, gender, age, or disabilities have led either to the mis- or underdevelopment of people's capabilities. Such corrections for the effects of unfair social practices are needed to make sure that competition is truly fair to all and not just fair in name only. For example, our system of compulsory public education and programs like Head Start use public resources (albeit in a highly imperfect way) to correct for inequalities in social advantage and to promote equality of opportunity.

Fair equality of opportunity does not require that opportunity be equal for all persons. It requires only that it be equal for persons with similar skills and talents, provided that people have had a fair chance to develop those talents and skills. The general principle of fair equality of opportunity does not imply leveling all individual differences in capabilities. These differences act as a baseline constraint on the degree to which the opportunities of individuals are truly equal. Our talents and skills and other capabilities vary, and ignoring these variations would be a highly inefficient way to organize society. If we ignored these variations, all of us—each of us— might be much worse off.

In theory, however, we can take advantage of the social productivity the natural distribution of capabilities permits while still mitigating the natural arbitrariness of that distribution (Rawls 1971). To do so, we must make appropriate transfers of social goods, such as income and other kinds of aid, to those with the least marketable talents and skills. In this way, we may all benefit from the results of social cooperation, even in ways justifiable to those who are fare less well. Within a more general account of social justice, unequal chances of success that derive from unequal talents may thus be compensated for in other ways in order to arrive at fair terms of cooperation among people of all levels of talents and skills.

This is hardly a complete account of social justice or fairness. There is, for example, controversy—in theory and in our society—about what other principles of distributive justice should govern transfers of social goods to those with poor life prospects. Still, (fair) equality of opportunity remains a central, widely held American ideal. Though our social practice often falls short of full compliance with this ideal, this is an area of our public life in which we have made visible moral progress over the last century.

Our ideas about equality of opportunity also commit us, as a matter of fairness and justice, to specific features of the design of our health care system. We want to emphasize from the outset, however, that not everyone will agree with the particular foundations we offer. Others may agree with many of our conclusions about fairness in health care reform but do so from other perspectives. (We return to these points later.) Our claim is not that we provide the only foundation for thinking about fairness in health care. We claim only to provide a reasonably comprehensive and coherent view that links these concerns to a central value in American life.

Equal Opportunity and the Importance of Health Care

What is the relationship between equal opportunity and the provision of health care services?

To answer this question, we need to ask some more basic questions about what health care does for us and what roles it plays in our lives. In fact, health care can do many things: it can extend our lives through prevention or cure; it can restore or prevent further loss of mental or physical function; it can harm or kill us; it can provide us with information and assurance about our bodies and ourselves; it can reduce pain and suffering. In different ways, by preventing or treating disease and disability, health care can keep us functioning as close to normal as possible. This is the central function of all forms of health care in our lives, whether public health, medical, preventive, acute, or chronic care (Daniels 1985), and it is the key function to keep in mind when considering justice in the delivery of health care.

Health care technologies can, of course, be used in other ways as well. Some medical technologies are used to enhance otherwise normal functioning or appearance, as in cosmetic (as opposed to reconstructive) uses of plastic surgery. But the uses of health care that most of us believe we are obliged to make available to others are uses that maintain or restore normal functioning, not simply any use that enhances our welfare. We reasonably consider this limited obligation in our public and private insurance practices, which, for example, do not cover cosmetic surgery. This distinction between the *treatment* of disease and disability and the *enhancement* of otherwise normal appearance or capabilities is reflected in the health care benefit packages of nearly every national health insurance system, whether public or mixed, around the world.

Why should it seem so important—so morally important—to protect normal functioning through the provision of health care services? The answer lies in this central fact: disease or dysfunction restrict access to life's opportunities. This is true whether they simply shorten our lives or they impair our ability to function, including through pain and suffering. Health care thus contributes to protecting our opportunities by protecting our functional capabilities. Since we are complex social creatures, our functional capabilities include our capabilities for normal emotional and cognitive functioning and not just physical capabilities.

The opportunities health care protects must be thought of more broadly than they are construed in our equal opportunity legislation. It is not just our opportunities to gain access to education, jobs, or offices that we seek to safeguard but also our opportunities to carry out the kinds of goals or tasks in life that all reasonable people may want to pursue, including engaging in meaningful social interaction with friends, family and colleagues; carrying out the tasks of daily living, including the bearing and raising of children; and engaging in avocations, including creative and recreational pursuits.

By aiming to keep us functioning normally, health care aims to preserve for us the range of opportunities we would have, were we not ill or disabled, given our talents and skills. In this way, it functions much like compensatory education services: these aim to correct for unfair social practices that lead to the underdevelopment of capabilities. They restore to us the range of capabilities—and thus opportunities—we would have had if those unfair practices had not interfered. Compensatory education programs and special education programs for the learning disabled, like health care services, thus draw justification from a commitment to fair, and not merely formal equality of opportunity. Fair equality of opportunity, unlike formal equality of opportunity, imposes a positive obligation on us to help people develop their capabilities despite a background of unfair social practices and the combined social and natural causes of disease and disability. A commitment to fair equality of opportunity thus recognizes that we should not allow people's prospects in life to be governed by correctable, morally arbitrary, or irrelevant differences between them, including those that result from disease and disability (see also Daniels 1996). By designing a health care system that keeps *all* people as close as possible to normal functioning, given reasonable resource constraints, we can in one important way fulfill our moral and legal obligations to protect equality of opportunity.

Limits on the Goals of Health Care

In explaining the relationship between equal opportunity and health care, we mentioned three points that deserve more comment. First, there is an important analogy between health care and education. Both are strategically important contributors to fair equality of opportunity. Both address needs that are not equally distributed among individuals. Various social factors, such as race, class, and family background, may produce special learning needs; so too may natural factors, such as the broad class of learning disabilities. To the extent that education is aimed at providing fair equality of opportunity, provision must be made to meet these special needs. Thus educational needs, like health care needs, differ from other basic needs, such as the need for food and clothing, which are more equally distributed among persons. The combination of their unequal distribution and their strategic importance for opportunity puts these needs in a separate category from those basic needs we can expect people to purchase from their fair income shares, like food and shelter. Both at the national level and in many states, legislation to meet special educational needs exists and is justified by reference to the opportunities it protects. Our account thus suggests another reason for thinking that American values and institutions should be able to provide support for a fair system of health care delivery.

This comparison to education also means that health care, however compelling, is not the only important social good. It competes with education, job training, and job creation, among other priorities, for social resources. Our commitments to meeting health care needs must thus be tempered by the fact that we must protect equality of opportunity in many different ways with resources that are limited. This account does not imply that health care is a bottomless pit.

A second point is the limited nature of the contribution that we think health care should make toward equality. We have suggested that health care aims at keeping people close to normal functioning and that doing so is part of what is required if the competition among people for success in life is to be a fair one. Equality of opportunity, as we understand it in our society, does not involve eliminating all individual differences. It commits us to judging people by morally relevant characteristics, such as their talents and skills, and this implies that we accept as a reasonable baseline the natural distribution of such capabilities. We correct for some "natural" effects on that distribution—disease and disability—but we do not attempt to eliminate all differences in the name of a radically expansive view of equal opportunity. The limited goal we ascribe to health care is that it helps us to be *normal* but not strictly *equal* competitors for success in life (see Daniels 1990a; Sabin and Daniels 1994). This limited goal thus conforms to our general understanding of the scope of the notion of equality of opportunity.

Some philosophers have argued that, despite our common beliefs, we are really committed to a more radical view of the demands of equality and of equality of opportunity, one that would dramatically expand the scope of our obligations in medicine. For example, some argue that we owe each other assistance whenever we lack, through no fault or choice of our own, the opportunity to enjoy equal welfare with others (Arneson 1988; Cohen 1989). Others argue that we should be concerned about inequality whenever the things we can do or be are not equal to those of others (Sen 1990, 1992). We sidestep this important disagreement here (but see Daniels 1990a; Rawls 1993; and Sabin and Daniels 1994), noting that concerns about *equality,* which are the focus of Arneson's, Cohen's, and Sen's discussions, are only part of an account of what justice or fairness requires. A full account of justice or fairness also must integrate our concerns about equality with consideration of efficiency and social productivity, as well as our concerns about liberty (see Cohen 1995). Our common view of equality of opportunity already includes these broader concerns, and that is why it seems less demanding and expansive than more radical interpretations (Daniels 1990a). We also sidestep speculation about the uses to which we might be obliged to put new medical technologies if we developed ways to alter genetically the distribution of human capabilities (see Buchanan, Brock, Daniels, and Wikler 1996).

A third point is that we have used, but not explained, the problematic notion of "normal functioning" and the related notions of disease and disability. For our purposes in designing a practical tool for assessing the fairness of reform, we do not have to resolve many philosophical disputes that arise concerning the concept of disease. For example, we do not have to resolve the question whether the concept of "disease" is an "objective" biomedical concept or a "social construct," reflecting value judgments that might vary from society to society.

Our account actually leaves room for elements of both views. We think of disease and disability as departures from normal functional organization and functioning for a typical member of our species, although we are aware that it is difficult to give a completely adequate philosophical account of the concept of function needed here (see Daniels 1985). Still, on this biomedical view, the intuitive idea is that we can study normal and abnormal function as objectively as the biomedical sciences allow. We thus reject the idea that a disease is simply any unwanted condition, even though historically societies have mistakenly called unwanted or undesirable conditions "diseases" when they were not. For example, masturbation was called a disease in the nineteenth century (Engelhardt 1974), but this did not make it a disease any more than calling whales "fish" made them fish. Since we believe that health is a distinct concept from happiness, we also reject the overly broad view of health as a "state of complete physical, mental, and social well-being, and not merely the absence of disease or infirmity," that is embodied in the World Health Organization definition (WHO 1946).

At the same time, our account allows for "social construction." In some cases there will be considerable controversy surrounding how to categorize human variation; the interaction of political and scientific views, for example, played an important role in the shifting categorization of homosexuality in psychiatric manuals two decades ago (see Bayer 1981). Different diseases and disabilities impair the range of our capabilities and opportunities differently. How important it is to treat them should reflect facts about their effects on the opportunities open to us, and this is clearly a matter of social interpretation. Similarly, the range of opportunities open to an individual is not just a function of facts about the individual's capabilities; it is also affected by general facts about a society, including its technological development, general wealth, and social structure. As a result, the same disease or disability may have different importance in different societies. For example, dyslexia may not be as important to address in an illiterate society as it is in the United States. Social construction plays a role here as well.

What Is Our Right to Health Care?

Some people fear that recognizing a right to health care allows people to "hijack" society with an endless list of claims to services as a "right" (Fried 1969; Engelhardt 1986). Even trying to restrict the right to health care can seem problematic: Will not people "need" everything that medical technology can do for them (Callahan 1987)? Will not every preference or demand for health care count as a need and every refusal be cast as a denial of rights?

By making the right to health care a special case of rights to equality of opportunity, we arrive at a reasonable, albeit incomplete and imperfect, way of restricting its scope while still recognizing its importance. Our account does not give individuals a basic right to have all of their health care needs met. At the same time, there are social obligations to design a health care system that protects opportunity through an appropriate set of services. If social obligations to provide appropriate health care are not met, then individuals are definitely wronged. For example, if people are denied access—because of discrimination or inability to pay—to a basic tier of services adequate to protect normal functioning, injustice is done to them. If the basic tier available to people omits important categories of services without consideration of their effects on normal functioning, for example, whole categories of mental health or long-term care or preventive services, their rights are violated.

Still, not every medical need gives rise to an entitlement to services. The scope and limits of rights to health care, that is, the entitlements they actually carry with them, will be relative to certain facts about a given system. For example, a health care system can protect opportunity only within the limits imposed by resource scarcity and technological development within a society. We cannot make a direct inference from the fact that an individual has a right to health care to the conclusion that this person is entitled to some specific health care service, even if the service would meet a health care need. Rather the individual is entitled to a specific service only if, in light of facts about a society's technological capabilities and resource limitations, it should be a part of a system that appropriately protects fair equality of opportunity.

Our account thus imposes important limits on the scope of a right to health care. The health care we have strongest claim to is care that *effec-*

tively promotes normal functioning by reducing the impact of disease and disability, thus protecting the range of opportunities that would otherwise be open to us. Words like "function" and "opportunity" have been given more precise meaning and measurement in recent years by the effort to measure health outcomes. They include the ability to carry out physical and mental activities, to carry out social functions and roles, to be free from pain, and to be in reasonably good spirits (Patrick and Erickson 1993).

This approach gives us a way of restricting the notion of "health care need" and a basis for making decisions about which needs are most important to meet. Although we may want medical services that can enhance our appearance, like cosmetic (as opposed to reconstructive) plastic surgery, or that can optimize our otherwise normal functioning, like some forms of counseling or some uses of Prozac, we do not truly need these services. We are obliged to help others achieve normal functioning, but we do not "owe" each other whatever it takes to make us more beautiful, strong, or completely happy (Daniels 1985). Even services that are aimed at treating disease and disability must be reasonably effective at doing so. What counts as "reasonably effective" is a matter of judgment and depends on the kind of condition and the consequences of not correcting it. But we do not owe people a chance to obtain miracles through whatever unproven procedures they prefer to try.

Even when some health care service is reasonably effective at meeting a medical need, not all such needs are equally important. When a disease or disability has little impact on the range of opportunities open to someone, it is not as morally important to treat as other conditions that more seriously impair opportunity. The effect on opportunity thus gives us some guidance in thinking about resource allocation priorities.

Unfortunately, impact on our range of opportunities gives only a crude and incomplete measure of the importance or priority we should put on a need or service. In making decisions about priorities for purposes of resource allocation in health care, we face difficult questions of distributive fairness that are not answered by this measure of importance. For example, we must sometimes make a choice between investing in a technology that delivers a significant benefit to few people or one that delivers a more modest benefit to a larger number of people. Sometimes we must make a choice between investing in a service that helps the sickest, most impaired patients or one that helps those whose functioning is less impaired. Sometimes we must decide between the fairness of giving a scarce resource to those who derive the largest benefit or giving a broader range of people some chance at getting a benefit. In all of these cases, we lack clear principles for deciding how to make our choices, and our account does not provide those principles either (Daniels 1993). In any health care system, then, some choices will have to be made by a fair, publicly accountable decision-making process. Our rights are not violated if the choices that are made in this way turn out to be ones that do not happen to meet our personal needs but instead meet the needs of others.

We commented in the previous section that health care is not the only important social good. It is not even the only way of protecting opportunity, and it competes for resources with other ways of doing so, like education. Reasonable limits must be set on health care resources, and we must carefully consider costs in making decisions about which health care needs are most important to meet. Failing to make careful, fair decisions of this sort will be unfair to patients whose more urgent or important needs are then not met. This said, in the American system the first priority before rationing anything is to reduce the extraordinary amount of overpayment, profit, and waste (perhaps a third of all expenditures) that keeps the United States from assuring its people ready access to all needed services like most other affluent countries. It would be a violation of our rights to health care if services that clearly promote normal functioning are unavailable in the system because waste and inefficiency consume valuable resources.

How equal must our rights to health care be? Specifically, must everyone receive exactly the same kinds of health care services and coverage, or is fairness in health care compatible with a "tiered" system? Around the world, even countries that offer universal health insurance differ in their answers to this question. In Canada and Norway, for example, no supplementary insurance is permitted. Everyone is served solely by the national health insurance schemes, though people who seek additional services or more rapid service may go elsewhere, as some Canadians do by crossing the border. In Britain, supplementary private insurance allows about 10 percent of the population to gain quicker access to services for which there is extensive queuing in the public system. Basing a right to health care on an obligation to protect equality of opportunity is compatible with the sort of tiering the British have, but it does not require it, and it imposes some constraints on the kind of tiering allowed.

The primary social obligation is to assure everyone access to a tier of services that effectively promotes normal functioning and thus protects equality of opportunity. Since health care is not the only important good, resources to be invested in the basic tier are appropriately and reasonably limited, for example, by democratic decisions about how much to invest in education or job training as opposed to health care. Because of their high "opportunity costs," there will be some beneficial medical services that it will be reasonable not to provide in the basic tier, or to provide only on a limited basis, for example with queuing. To say that these services have "high opportunity costs" means that providing them consumes resources that would produce greater health benefits and protect opportunity more if used in other ways.

In a society that permits significant income and wealth inequalities, some people will want to buy coverage for these additional services. Why not let them? After all, we allow people to use their after-tax income and wealth as they see fit to pursue the "quality of live" and opportunities they prefer. The rich can buy special security systems for their homes, safer cars, and private schooling for their children. Why not allow them to buy supplementary health care for their families?

One objection to allowing a supplementary tier is that its existence might undermine the basic tier either economically or politically. It might attract better quality providers away from the basic tier, or raise costs in the basic tier, reducing the ability of society to meet its social obligations. The supplementary tier might weaken political support for the basic tier, for example, by undercutting the social solidarity needed if people are to remain committed to ensuring opportunity for all. These objections are serious, and where a supplementary tier takes away from the basic tier either economically or politically, priority must be given to protecting the basic tier. In principle, however, it seems possible to design a system in which the supplementary tier does not undermine the basic one. If that can be done, then a system that permits tiering avoids restricting liberty in ways that some find seriously objectionable.

A second objection is to the structure of inequality that results from tiering. Compare two scenarios. In one, most people are adequately served by the basic tier and only the best-off groups in society have the means and see the need to purchase supplementary insurance. That is the case in Great Britain. In the other, the basic tier serves only the poorest groups in society and most other people buy supplementary insurance. The Oregon plan to expand Medicaid eligibility partly through rationing the services it covers has aspects of this structure of inequality, since most people are covered by plans that avoid these restrictions (Daniels 1991). The first scenario seems preferable to the second on grounds of fairness. In the second, the poorest groups can complain that they are left behind by others in society even in the protection of their health. In the first, the majority has less grounds for reasonable resentment or regret.

If the basic tier is not undermined by higher tiers and if the structure of the inequality that results is not objectionable, then it is difficult to see why some tiering should not be allowed. There is a basic conflict here between concerns about equality and concerns about liberty, between wanting to make sure everyone is treated properly with regard to health care and wanting to give people the liberty to use their (after-tax) resources to improve their lives as they see fit. In practice, the crucial constraint on the liberty we allow people seems to depend on the magnitude of the benefit available in the supplementary tier and unavailable in the basic tier. Highly visible forms of saving lives and improving function would be difficult to exclude from the basic tier while we make them available in a supplementary tier. In principle, however, some forms of tiering will not be unfair even when they involve medical benefits not available to everyone.

Other Perspectives on Fairness

We have suggested that widely held American values, especially a determination to protect equality of opportunity, provide reasonable foundations for thinking about fairness or justice in health care. Equal opportunity provides a basis for a right to health care, but it also helps us set reasonable limits on the entitlements that come with such a right. It does not turn a right to health care into a bottomless pit.

Our suggestion provides some antidote to claims that Americans are too individualistic to support comprehensive health care reform. But the antidote is not a complete cure. There remains considerable controversy in the United States about the scope and content of our commitments to equality of opportunity, just as there is controversy about what fairness in health care reform requires. The current debate about affirmative action is in part a controversy about our commitments to equality of opportunity. Because of this controversy, our view might be criticized as disguised "ideology" or "politics masquerading as ethics." After commenting briefly about some of these issues, we suggest how our use of the benchmarks that we developed avoids this accusation.

We have come to see the provision of equality of opportunity as a requirement of justice in our society for many reasons and from many divergent perspectives. Nevertheless, it is worth noting that some recent work in the theory of justice supports this outcome. Rawls (1971) proposed that the way to discover the fundamental principles of justice is to make us choose principles from behind a "veil of ignorance" that keeps us from knowing what our individual traits are and where we will end up in life. This stipulation forces us to make rules that we would have to live by and find acceptable regardless of whether we were a fifty-eight-year-old Chicano farmhand with progressive arthritis and a large family or an eight-year-old mildly retarded daughter of professional parents. We want provisions and rules that would be fair regardless who we turn out to be.

On this view, the principles we would choose correct for many natural characteristics and social contingencies that seem arbitrary from a moral perspective. We would include basic liberties of the sort provided in our Constitution. We would insist that fair equality of opportunity be guaranteed, and we would not accept inequalities in income or wealth that did not work to the advantage of those who are worst off, because we might turn out to be among the worst off. Fair terms of social cooperation, however, do not require that all inequalities be eliminated or that we ignore the fact that talents and skills are not equally distributed. In fact, a well-designed society will capitalize on the unequal distribution of talents and skills to generate more resources and wealth than an equal distribution would allow, so that the smallest shares of the larger social pie are larger than would be equal shares of a smaller pie. Fairness requires that we must make the social structure work in ways that are acceptable even from the perspective of those who are worst off.

The political liberalism articulated by Rawls is not the only framework of values that can support the sorts of commitments reflected in the benchmarks we develop. The point might be illustrated by an anecdote from the ill-fated history of President Clinton's Health Care Task Force. The task force included an Ethics Working Group, composed of a diverse set of bioethicists, including physicians, lawyers, theologians, and philosophers. The group was asked to articulate principles and values that should underlie the Clinton proposal (see the preface and also Brock and Daniels 1994; Daniels 1994).

When members of the group deliberated about foundational issues, they could agree on little. Some were comfortable talking about "rights" and "entitlements" to health care. Others found this framework too individualistic and not focused enough on the idea of community and mutual caring. When the group discussed the specific principles and values, however, it was able to agree on a dozen principles and values that should characterize health care reform (White House Domestic Policy Council 1993). Whereas some used the language of political liberalism to talk about limits to our rights and the importance of efficiency, others used more religiously laden terminology, preferring, for example, to talk about the "stewardship" of community resources. The group also discovered that clarifying how the principles translated into features of the system required distinguishing agreements about values from agreements and disagreements about economic and political institutions. This analytic task facilitated discussion. It often defused what began as heated moral disagreements, converting them into apparently more tractable disagreements, for example, about the feasibility of regulating a practice in a particular way.

Of course, the Ethics Working Group did not represent the full spectrum of American views about values or the workings of markets and governments. Had more of its members been proponents of highly libertarian perspectives, for instance, the group might not have reached agreement that universal coverage was a requirement of fair reform. Libertarians, for example, might not even support government regulation to protect formal equality of opportunity: that would be seen as interference with more fundamental rights of contract (see Nozick 1974). More moderate libertarians might accept legislation protecting formal equality of opportunity, but they would see protection of fair equality of opportunity as an unacceptable transfer of resources. Libertarians would also have objected to compulsory individual coverage as well as to employer mandates, for both restrict the liberty of individuals to form contracts as they see fit. Libertarians would furthermore not agree in principle with any tax-subsidized transfers to make coverage for the poor possible. In their view, the power to impose taxes coercively in order to pursue social goals exceeds the legitimate authority of the state, since it violates basic property rights of individuals. Others, who strongly resemble libertarians in their conclusions about minimal government, argue that we should seek private as opposed to public solutions to problems because they are more efficient, not because they better preserve liberty.

By resting our benchmarks on one central American value, fair equality of opportunity, we have thus not eliminated all sources of moral disagreement within American culture. Nor have we singled out the only framework of values that can be used to justify these as benchmarks of fairness. We have, however, provided a coherent foundation that is consistent with some of our most deeply held American values. That is not the same as assuring consensus and guaranteeing that our account of fairness will be justifiable to everyone, regardless of their beliefs. Most importantly, we are not trying to "seize" the moral high ground by appropriating the term "fairness" and justifying our political goals by appeal to it. As a justification for features of reform, the matrix we develop will have only limited force, for it will be accepted as relevant only by those who accept its underlying assumptions.

The primary function of our benchmarks for fairness is analytic, not justificatory. It helps us locate points of disagreement and agreement so that we can see whether the disagreements are fundamentally traceable to basic disagreements about moral principles or values, or they stem from disagreements about nonmoral or empirical issues, such as the workings of institutions and their effects on people. Conclusions about whether features of a system or institution promote fairness rest on *both* moral and empirical beliefs. Our matrix should facilitate discussion of what features produce fairness even where there is both moral and empirical disagreement. It is intended to put issues of fairness on the table and to force constructive dialogue about them.

From Fairness to Benchmarks

For the most part, we have talked about access to health care *services* because that is what really matters. Insurance is merely a means to this end.

People do not "want insurance" because they think insurance is itself valuable. They want health insurance only so that health care can be accessible when it is needed. Many universal health care systems do not have what is properly called insurance. They have prepaid health care budgets that they call "health insurance." If a nation has a system for gathering funds in order to pay for health care (or highways), it is not "insurance" in the traditional sense. This is particularly the case when the so-called insurance pays for many routine expenses rather than for uncommon, large, and unpredictable losses. The point here is that preoccupations with "national health insurance" and how it is structured should not distract us from the central goal: to provide equal access to needed and effective health care.

We have organized the dimensions of fairness in health care into ten benchmarks. Some of the benchmarks derive directly from the equal opportunity account of fairness we have used, and our discussion provides a clear rationale for them. Others draw on aspects of fairness that we have not discussed in detail, for example, the widely held view that the richer we are, the better we can afford to bear the burden of financing general social obligations. These views are by no means uncontroversial in our society. Proposals for a "flat tax" to replace the more progressive income tax are being discussed seriously in some quarters, though they are defended for their "simplicity" rather than for their fairness, and they are attacked for their unfairness. In building some of these views about fairness into the benchmarks, we do not intend to hide our assumptions. Rather we make them explicit so that they can become the focus of constructive discussion about the design of reform proposals.

The first two benchmarks measure universal access, one focusing on financial barriers and the other on nonfinancial barriers. If access to services is not universal, then equality of opportunity is weakened. If access is not universal, other morally irrelevant social contingencies—income and wealth, education level, or geographical location—will determine access to health care, not medical need.

Fairness, as we have construed it, also requires that the criteria for inclusion of health care services in a benefit package are their effectiveness and relative importance in protecting opportunity through promoting normal functioning. The benchmark measuring comprehensiveness of benefits employs that criterion, prohibiting, for example, categorical exclusions of preventive or mental health or other types of services without regard for their effect on normal functioning. Such exclusions are a common feature of many current insurance plans. The uniformity component of the benchmark assures that significant inequalities in the protection of opportunity are not built into benefit packages.

By treating fairness in health care as a special case of promoting equality of opportunity, we emphasize that it is a social obligation we must all share.

Table 2-1.   Benchmarks of Fairness for National Health
Care Reform

Benchmark 1: Universal Access—Coverage and Participation
Benchmark 2: Universal Access—Minimizing Nonfinancial Barriers
Benchmark 3: Comprehensive and Uniform Benefits
Benchmark 4: Equitable Financing—Community-Rated Contributions
Benchmark 5: Equitable Financing—By Ability to Pay
Benchmark 6: Value for Money—Clinical Efficacy
Benchmark 7: Value for Money—Financial Efficiency
Benchmark 8: Public Accountability
Benchmark 9: Comparability
Benchmark 10: Degree of Consumer Choice

The benchmarks requiring community-rated premiums and out-of-pocket payments that are means-based specify two aspects of the fair sharing of the burdens of meeting those obligations. Community rating means that health status differences among individuals will not determine the cost of health care insurance. Means-based payments assure that all medical bills are proportional to the ability to pay. The claim that we should pay for our general social obligations according to our ability to pay, such as through a progressive tax structure, clearly goes beyond the concept of fair equality of opportunity.

Four benchmarks focus on certain limits to society's obligations to protect opportunity through the delivery of health care. The comparability benchmark reminds us that health care is not the only important social good: other services, like education, have a profound impact on opportunity, and other uses of social resources, for national defense and the criminal justice system, promote security and protect our liberties. The two "value for money" benchmarks emphasize the ways in which a proposal must strive to get rid of wasteful uses of health care dollars. It might seem that elimination of waste was really not an issue of fairness and should not show up as a benchmark. If a system is wasteful, however, and resources are limited, then the needs of some will be sacrificed to wasteful features of the system. Their opportunities will not be as well protected as in a less wasteful system, and they will be wronged. Thus, eliminating waste and securing value for money is a matter of fairness. But even if all waste were corrected, advances in medical technology demand that hard choices be made about which beneficial uses of medical services are most important. This prescribes a benchmark concerning public accountability through fair procedures for making such decisions. Justice quite generally requires that the grounds for making decisions that affect our lives in fundamental ways be accessible to us.

The tenth benchmark concerns choice. This is a complex issue since there are many dimensions to choice: treatments, physicians, insurance plans. It may not be possible to maximize choice along all these dimensions at once, and some kinds of choice compromise other benchmarks of fairness. For example, a choice between insurance plans with different levels and ranges of benefits can deeply compromise community rating and equal access.

Most of the benchmarks are multidimensional themselves. Performance on a benchmark is determined by the average score for several criteria. These criteria are a way of making explicit some of our assumptions about fairness; they are a necessary complexity. They are also a way to clarify some of our empirical assumptions, such as our assumptions about how institutions, both public and private, work. In the benchmarks concerning "value for money," assumptions about the complexity and cost of administering some insurance schemes play a key role in scoring. If these assumptions are wrong or controversial, they should become a focus of candid discussion. Our point is to show how these assumptions, combined with a concern to obtain value for money in protecting opportunity, yield conclusions about the fairness of the system or proposal for reform. Our matrix does not arbitrarily coopt the concept of fairness for political purposes but provides an analytic structure that can clarify public debate.

Although these benchmarks draw on an underlying account of fairness that emphasizes equality of opportunity, we think there can be considerable agreement on them even without appeal to that account because the benchmarks capture widely shared values in our society. People may hold some or all of those values without combining them into a theoretical framework exactly like the one we describe. It seemed important to show that the matrix had the coherence provided by that underlying account, even if it can be used by people who accept its value on more pragmatic grounds. Finally, the matrix does not capture every aspect of the moral assessment of health care delivery. We concentrate on issues of fairness but leave aside some other important matters, including, for example, the respect for professional integrity of clinicians. In developing this matrix, we do not preclude the development of a more comprehensive one.

3

Benchmarks of Fairness

The benchmarks described in this chapter are intended to enhance deliberation about fairness, putting it centrally in the debate about reform. They form an analytic tool for thinking about the fairness of different aspects of health care reform. They are most useful for disentangling the complex moral and empirical assumptions that underlie our judgments and disagreements about the key dimensions of fairness. They will not produce immediate agreement on the relative fairness of alternatives, in part because they embody particular assumptions that not everyone accepts. By being explicit about these assumptions, they aim to improve debate and understanding about fairness, not to end it by stipulation.

There is an unavoidable complexity to the benchmarks because what they measure is complex. For example, the concept of "access" to needed and effective treatments may have seemed simple or straightforward when we used it in the previous chapter, but there are many obstacles to access and therefore many ways for access to services to fail. Reform proposals may address some of these problems and not others, making relative success or fairness multidimensional. As a result, most of the benchmarks involve a cluster of related elements and require more than one criterion.

Further complication arises because different kinds of rationales are needed for different criteria. Some criteria derive fairly directly from the equal opportunity framework, others from other aspects of fairness. Still others depend on economic, sociological, or political beliefs. For example, benchmark 1, concerning insurance coverage aspects of universal access, includes as a criterion the portability and continuity of coverage. If health care coverage is to promote normal functioning, and through it equality of opportunity, as suggested in chapter 2, access to services must not be jeopardized when we change jobs or geographical areas. Although this criterion has its rationale in the underlying account of fairness, it also has salience because the vagaries of our employment-based system of coverage have made these issues a matter of concern to millions of Americans. In other cases, issues of fairness other than equality of opportunity bear on the selection of the criterion. For example, part of the rationale for making coverage mandatory is that we thus prevent some people from free-loading on the willingness of others to contribute.

In other cases, empirical considerations are part of the rationale for inclusion of the criterion. For example, we appeal to the cost-containment advantages of universal coverage in defending a rapid phase-in of universal coverage (see the later discussion of benchmark 1). It is important to understand just how differing empirical assumptions affect conclusions about fairness. Contrast the following two arguments:

Phase-in contingent on savings is unfair.

1. Fairness requires universal coverage as quickly as feasible.
2. Phase-in is feasible only if it can be financed.
3. *A phase-in period with nonuniversal coverage reduces the ability to contain costs in the system because of continued cost shifting.*
4. Reduced cost containment means some people will remain uncovered longer than necessary.
5. A system with phase-in contingent on savings is less fair than one without that contingency.

Phase-in contingent on savings is not unfair.

1. Fairness requires universal coverage as quickly as is feasible.
2. Phase-in is feasible only if it can be financed.
3. *A phase-in period with nonuniversal coverage has little effect on the ability to contain costs in the system.*
4. People will not remain uncovered longer than necessary with a phase-in contingent on savings.
5. A system with phase-in contingent on savings is not less fair than one without that contingency.

These two arguments differ in their premise 3, which makes a claim about how cost containment will work and its implications. There may be little disagreement on values between the advocates of the two arguments. The value premises (1) are identical. But the conclusions (5) about fairness differ. Since the criteria for our benchmarks require conclusions about fairness, they will be sensitive to different assumptions about economic, sociological, and political matters. (By "assumptions" here and later, we do not mean to suggest there is no support or evidence for these claims: they may be well supported by research and widely believed. We use "assumption" to identify a starting point for an argument or analysis.) It is unavoidable that judgments about fairness depend on such varied factors. Disagreements about fairness may depend on differences in values, but they may depend on these other differences as well.

Being explicit and clear about this complexity and its sources is part of what makes this matrix useful as an analytic tool. We make no pretense to have "gotten it right" in all the assumptions we make. Nor is our goal the "truth about fairness, once and for all." Our goal is to produce a useful tool for framing the debate about fairness of reform, and tools are not true or false, only more or less useful. Attempts to use the matrix will stimulate debate and lead to modifications, improvements, and hopefully to better understanding. Ideally the tool will facilitate better reform.

Benchmark 1: Universal Access—Coverage and Participation

Any fair health care system must make a reasonable array of needed and effective health care services available to everyone regardless of their health conditions, risks, or ability to pay. Generally, this means that public insurance or some combination of public and private insurance must include everyone and provide that reasonable array of benefits. What makes the benefits "reasonable" is a complex function of the importance of the health care needs they meet, their effectiveness, judgments about the relative importance of health care services and other social goods, and other facts about a society's wealth, technological development, and social structure. This basic principle about *universal access* and thus *universal inclusion in an insurance scheme* follows directly from the equal opportunity account (though there are other ways of supporting it as well). We return to what services are reasonably included in our discussion of benchmark 3 and other aspects of universal access in our discussion of benchmark 2; here we concentrate on how the insurance scheme works to ensure access.

We distinguish three aspects of universal inclusion: the proportion of the population included and whether their participation is mandatory; how quickly universal inclusion is achieved; and how flexibly and effectively the scheme provides access through changes in jobs and living conditions. Each aspect is made the subject of a separate criterion. A reform proposal that fails to include everyone, that slowly expands inclusion, or that impedes portability or continuity of coverage is less fair than one that performs better on these measures of inclusion.

A direct appeal to the equal opportunity account underlies each of these three criteria, for reasons that are obvious. We noted the implication of the underlying account for portability and continuity above. Other considerations of fairness and some nonmoral considerations also contribute to the rationale for these criteria, and we want to be explicit about these. We have labeled the first criterion "mandatory coverage and participation," and we want to explain why we insist, on grounds of fairness, that the inclusion be mandatory. It might seem to some that if society provides the opportunity for universal access, but some people prefer not to participate, then we should allow them that liberty. Coercing people into participation, some might object, violates certain rights or liberties.

Our criterion assumes that requiring participation is fair, all things considered. In our society, people who "choose" to remain uninsured are generally provided with medical services, especially on an emergency basis. Even people who insist they would refuse services that they did not pay for may change their minds when faced with immediate needs; or they may not be competent to express their wishes when the services are provided. Those who exercise a liberty not to purchase voluntary insurance, perhaps because they believe they are at lower than average risk and that premiums are a poor bargain for them, will then impose costs on third parties who do support our system of medical services through their premiums and taxes. There is a "public good" argument here as well, since a system is less stable if it provides benefits to people who are "free" not to pay for them. Since the public good at issue here is extremely important, because health care protects equal opportunity, the obligation to contribute to its support is more important than any supposed liberty not to.

An issue that arose during recent discussions of health care reform was the speed with which the "phase-in" of reform, including universal coverage, was to take place. Some argued that universal coverage should be contingent on the reform saving enough money to finance expanded coverage. We think it is unfair to make coverage depend on such savings. The rationale for our inclusion of this criterion involves several different considerations. First, making inclusion depend on savings distributes the burdens of containing costs inequitably. The burden falls hardest—with serious health consequence—on those who continue without coverage during a long phase-in (Hadley, Steinberg, and Feder 1991; Franks, Clancy, and Gold 1993; Stoddard, Peter, and Newacheck 1994). Moreover, it is unclear when one has saved "enough" to "afford" wider coverage. Because medical expenditures constantly rise even in the most financially disciplined systems, one always has the excuse that not enough has been saved to afford greater universality. Third, lack of universal coverage makes cost containment more difficult, especially because it leads to cost shifting. Subordinating universality to cost containment, which has long been the American strategy, undermines the goal of cost containment and is a principal reason (along with the lack of a global health care budget) why costs in the United States have increased more rapidly than in countries with universal coverage. Fourth, putting cost containment before universal coverage invites payers to save money by reducing access or coverage even more than at present, especially for those who are the most sick and therefore need coverage the most. This is the "inverse coverage law" that one observes in voluntary competitive systems: those who need the most coverage are likely to get the least and to pay more for what they do get (Light 1992b).

In the United States, this inequality worsened during the 1980s as employers and health insurance companies contained *their* costs by shifting them to patients through such techniques as increased deductibles and co-payments, exclusions clauses, waiting periods, within-group underwriting, "gotcha clauses," policy terminations, payment caps, policy churning, and forms of claims harassment (Stone 1993; Light 1992b). These techniques not only discriminated against the sick, but they also failed to reduce the rapid increase in expenditures that plagued the economy during the 1970s, because they actually increased costs while they blocked effective forms of cost containment (Light 1992a). Thus for reasons of principle and practicality, universal coverage is the most fair and effective way to restrain health care costs.

An important boundary issue concerns the definition of "everyone" in the inclusion criterion. Should it include visitors, people who fly in from other countries for medical care, illegal residents, or other categories of people? This is a complex question that requires separate treatment, and we cannot consider it here. Fairness arguments, for example, will fall on both sides of the question about inclusion of illegal residents or for anyone who does not contribute to the support of the system.

Benchmark 2: Universal Access—Minimizing Nonfinancial Barriers

Universal health insurance for a comprehensive list of effective services does not necessarily guarantee equal or even reasonable access to them. It eliminates financial barriers to those services, but it does not eliminate other important barriers. Equitable access requires these four conditions be met:

1. appropriate resources, including personnel, equipment, and facilities, are where they are needed and are reachable by those who need them;
2. education and training are sufficient and appropriate to supply the needed personnel;

3. steps are taken to facilitate the use of services by people with different languages, cultures, and class backgrounds;
4. adequate education and information are provided to facilitate negotiation of the system.

The first two conditions affect the supply or availability of services; the second two, their use. We convert these conditions into criteria for evaluating benchmark 2.

Access requires the availability of services. Yet the availability of good public health, preventive, and medical services varies from state to state and town to town. More generally, since supply is influenced by demand, the fact that poor working people in urban or rural areas lack insurance leads over time to inequities in the availability of services. Some of the inequality in availability is affected by other factors as well and would persist even if universal access to insurance were assured. This means that making the supply and distribution of appropriate staff and the resources more equitable is as important as a universal health insurance card. Specific steps must be taken to alter the balance of people trained.

There are several other nonfinancial barriers to access besides availability. Transportation is another dimension affecting equitable access. It may vary from a bus or car ride to a helicopter service for the severely burned. Arrangements at work or home may also seriously impair access. People have lost their jobs for taking time to seek medical treatment, though taking time off can clearly be abused. Some home situations greatly impair the ability to leave for medical attention, even if the person has an insurance card, transportation, and a facility nearby.

Besides reducing physical barriers to access, reforms should also aim to reduce the barriers of language, culture, and social class. Efforts should be made to equalize people's understanding about health issues and information about health specific services. The general point is that equal access only begins with universal coverage. Scoring of this benchmark therefore centers on the degree to which a proposal details programs for minimizing maldistributions of resources and access barriers of culture, language, class, and information about access.

The primary rationale for the benchmark derives from our interest in protecting equal opportunity. An important set of assumptions about the workings of the medical market and its effects underlies the other criteria. Universal coverage would have some effects on the availability and distribution of resources: broader demand by previously underserved people will affect supply. These effects take time, and they work imperfectly. For example, vastly increasing the supply of physicians in the United States led to some dispersion of specialists to rural and underserved urban areas. The dispersion was inadequate to meet needs, took place slowly, and was accompanied by oversupply in areas already well served. Strong preferences of providers for suburban living conditions, for example, affect the cost and rate of dispersion. Different incentives in the educational and training system for personnel may work against or out of synchronization with market-based demands. Finally, markets may not be responsive to cultural and educational differences in our pluralist society.

Our account thus places less confidence than some would on the ability of a market with improved insurance coverage to produce an equitable redistribution of services, that is, a redistribution that adequately meets new demands and that reduces barriers to access in all four areas we have noted. We believe proposals must explicitly address these nonfinancial barriers if access is to be fair.

Benchmark 3: Comprehensive and Uniform Benefits

Fairness requires *equitable access to an appropriate set of health care services*. Fairness thus involves requirements on both *access* and *services*. Our first two benchmarks clarify what steps must be taken to assure that access is equitable. Benchmark 3 sets some general constraints on what counts as appropriate services. Specifically, there are three criteria for scoring this benchmark: How comprehensive are the benefits? Are there constraints on inequalities in benefits and quality due to tiering? Does the range of benefits depend on savings produced by reform? In large part, the rationale for these constraints derives directly from the underlying equal opportunity framework.

The central function of health care services is to keep us functioning as close to normal as possible. Since maintaining normal functioning protects the range of opportunities open to people, by providing an appropriate set of health care services, we make a significant contribution to protecting equality of opportunity. Health care services are not the only way of protecting opportunity, however, and opportunity is not the only fundamentally important good, so it is reasonable to limit resources we devote to health care (see benchmark 9). Decisions about these limits should be explicit and should be made in a publicly accountable way (see benchmark 8). When we talk about "comprehensive" benefits in this benchmark, then, we assume that reasonable limits will be set on what counts as comprehensive.

Two key ideas from our account of equal opportunity motivate the criteria relevant to this benchmark. First, the importance of including services in a benefit package depends on their relative contribution to the protection of equality of opportunity. This idea has a bearing on which reasons for excluding services are allowable. Second, we have obligations to protect everyone's opportunities. This has a bearing on what kinds of inequalities in benefits we think permissible in the health care system. We need to say more about each of these issues.

What kinds of reasons can we give for excluding services from a "fair" benefit package? Two generally acceptable reasons for excluding services are that they are not needed for the treatment or prevention of disease or disability (this is part of what is captured in the problematic terminology of "medical necessity"; Daniels and Sabin 1991), or that they are ineffective. Both reasons involve easy and hard cases. Some lines are fairly easily drawn, for example, between uses of plastic surgery for reconstruction after disease or trauma, which are arguably "medically necessary," and uses to enhance otherwise normal appearance or function, which are excludable (Daniels 1985). In other cases, such as in the provision of some mental health services, the boundary is harder to draw, though it is still possible to defend a reasonable boundary between "needed" treatments and merely "desired" enhancements (Sabin and Daniels 1994). In general, it is disturbing how many ways the profession expands the notion of "need" (Payer 1988, 1992; Conrad and Schneider 1992). Since difficult and controversial choices will have to be made, it is important that the procedures for making them be explicit and publicly accountable (see benchmark 8).

We may also exclude services if their effectiveness is refuted or has not yet been proven. To provide a scientific basis for these judgments, much research on outcomes and on the development of clinical guidelines must be done (Hadorn 1992). It is disturbing how many procedures continue to be performed even after evidence appears that they are ineffectual (see, for example, Fowler, Barry and Lu-Yao, 1993). In addition, a great proportion of medical interventions have not been systematically studied for their effectiveness at all. A properly designed system would take steps to close the gap between use and knowledge about effectiveness. Similarly, some effort must be made to assess the effectiveness of nontraditional therapies. Difficult questions lie in this area, because many patients believe in and are satisfied by therapies that might prove to have no measurable benefits aside from placebo effects. The principle of covering needed and effective care is much clearer than its application (Caplan 1987).

What kinds of reasons should we not permit for excluding services? One common practice in U.S. insurance is the categorical exclusion of whole areas of service, e.g., preventive, home care, or mental health services. A similar practice involves setting an arbitrary dollar ceiling on the use of services in a certain category. These types of exclusions or limits run counter to the fundamental idea that services be assessed for their impact on normal functioning and thereby on opportunities. Excluding whole categories of service simply because they are convenient for drawing administrative lines thus discriminates unfairly against people who need them. The lack of parity in our health insurance coverage for mental and physical illness, for example, ignores completely the effectiveness of many mental health services and the significant impact mental illness has on normal functioning and opportunity. Long-term care services, including home care services, are also much less available in American insurance policies than they should be given their impact on functioning or the degree to which they compensate for losses of functioning. Worries about the "moral hazard" of people claiming to need those services when they do not are not a reason for categorical exclusion of those services. Such problems can be addressed by case management techniques. The fundamental issue is whether we are being fair to people by meeting the full range of their needs.

The stand taken here in favor of comprehensiveness in the benefit package runs counter to the view that our moral obligations only involve our providing a "basic" or "bare bones" policy to the poorest members of society; others may then purchase more comprehensive plans as their "taste" for medical services requires. The problem with this approach is that the cost of the uncovered services accentuates the unequal distribution of both illness and income among social classes; the poor get sicker, and the sick get poorer. In addition, insurers or payers can easily exercise the "inverse coverage law" by discriminating against those with high risks, illness, or disabilities (Light 1992b). Thus the test for this benchmark is how the benefits for the most disadvantaged compare with those for the most advantaged. The opportunities of all must be protected in a fair system.

It is sometimes argued that a comprehensive benefits plan forces people to pay for benefits they do not need and for benefits that someone else needs. The "fair" approach, then, is to let people buy health insurance that includes only the benefits they want. This approach, however, has a couple of basic problems. First, people often do not know what services they will need. Much ill health is unpredictable, particularly in a family plan. Second, to the extent that different risk groups know who they are and what services they need, having each risk group pay for only their risks quickly leads to a steeply tiered market in which the sick must pay far more for the broader and deeper policies they need. The inverse coverage law manifests itself again, making health care unaffordable for the sick. In short, this argument against comprehensive benefits does not seem well thought out.

Beyond the comprehensive benefits, this benchmark leaves room for extra or tiered services. In principle, it does not prohibit individuals from purchasing supplemental insurance or paying directly for more elaborate services, so long as they do not undermine the basic package. However, the more extensive supplemental services become, the more discriminatory the system will become, and the more their presence will drive up costs as lesser plans feel pressure to keep up. This has happened among German insurance funds, even though they are community rated and have a comprehensive benefits package (Wysong and Abel 1990).

The criterion we propose treats a proposal as more fair than another if it has relatively less tiering and assures more uniformity in quality. The more tiering is restricted to amenities or services that have little impact on outcomes, the less problematic it is. A fair reform will aim to minimize the differences in quality of services and providers. Many developments today towards uniform standards and measurable differences in quality promise to make what services exist more fair across social groups.

We have included a separate criterion in this benchmark to address the relationship among the costs of comprehensive benefits, the savings generated by reform, and the scope of benefits permitted. The issue here is similar to the argument concerning phase-in of universal coverage: when should access to certain benefits for those unable to afford to buy additional coverage themselves depend on the reformed system generating savings sufficient to pay for the additional benefits? If savings sufficient to cover these services fail to materialize because of other problems in the design of the system, for instance, administrative or clinical inefficiency, then we are holding people with real medical needs hostage to our inability to reform the system in proper ways. This unfairness is captured by this criterion.

Benchmark 4: Equitable Financing—Community-rated Contributions

Fairness concerns not only the benefits we are obliged to provide— equitable access to an appropriate set of services—but how we share the burden of meeting that obligation. Benchmarks 4 and 5 address how these burdens are to be shared between the well and the ill, and among different income groups, respectively. We separate these issues into two benchmarks in part because a premium-based private insurance system has been such a prominent feature of our health care system and is retained in most reform proposals but also because they are logically distinct. A premium-based system could be community rated, satisfying the criteria for fairness of benchmark 4, but it would still fail to be as progressively financed as benchmark 5 requires, unless there was an income-based sliding scale for premiums. If, however, a system was financed through a progressive tax, then in effect it would be community rated (even though it is not premium based), since the cost of coverage would not reflect health risks but ability to pay. We shall return later to comment on one apparent paradox raised by community rating: in a community-rated, premium-based system, healthy but poor people may help subsidize the health care costs of sick but affluent people. This subsidy runs counter to the requirements of benchmark 5.

The appeal to fair equality of opportunity plays an important role in justifying both benchmarks 4 and 5. Because it provides a foundation for the claim that we have obligations to provide appropriate medical services to people who need them, it explains why we cannot simply treat the financing of insurance for these services in the same way we view payment for other kinds of insurance. Instead, we must share the burdens for this kind of insurance in the way we usually share the burdens of paying for our other social obligations. In our country, for example, minorities and the poor generally suffer disproportionately as victims of violent crime. We do not, however, think that they should pay more for police protection as a result. We think providing fundamental security of the person to all people is a social obligation for which we must all pay, and we generally finance such services through a broad tax on everyone.

Other considerations of fairness besides the appeal to equal opportunity also affect the rationale for benchmarks 4 and 5, however, and we shall have to see how these play a role in justifying the specific criteria involved in the two benchmarks. For example, we shall say more about the notion of ability to pay in our discussion of benchmark 5. We shall also reply shortly to the objection that we have no obligations to share the costs of health conditions people bring on themselves, so that premiums may legitimately reflect self-induced health risks.

First, however, we need to define "community rating" and explain why we support it on grounds of fairness rather than accepting the concept of "actuarial fairness," which forms the basis of other forms of private insurance. Actuarial fairness holds that people should pay premiums that reflect the actual levels of risk they face. The criteria for scoring benchmark 4 center on the degree to which a proposal gathers money independently, both directly or indirectly, of people's health risks (Light 1992b). One criterion requires that premiums themselves not reflect health risks but be based on the average costs of an insuree in as large an insurance pool as is possible, ideally the entire community. (Premiums might still reasonably vary from community to community in ways that reflect differences in health care costs by region.) This criterion would eliminate standard medical underwriting practices used by insurers for individual medical insurance policies and increasingly for small- and middle-sized group policies. Underwriting is the process through which insurers determine applicants' levels of risk in order to exclude those at high risk or who face a specific risk from coverage or to charge them nonstandard (usually higher) rates. The second criterion reduces other ways in which the sick are made to pay more for their coverage. It includes minimizing deductibles, co-payments, payment caps, waiting periods, and other "back-end" ways (as opposed to "front-end" premiums) of making the sick bear the burden of the costs of their illness.

Most countries prohibit medical underwriting or risk rating because it contradicts and obstructs one of the most important goals of the system: to help high-risk and sick people receive the services they need. In community rating, all people, regardless of their health risks, are treated alike. This means the healthier support the sicker, and when they become sick, others help them. Europeans refer to this as the solidarity principle, the idea that we all help each other in times of need. We have instead appealed to the principle of fair equality of opportunity to justify the same result. Either notion supplies us with a relevant conception of social fairness that is clearly distinct from the concept of actuarial fairness. Actuarial fairness, as we noted, holds that it is most fair for each risk group to pay only for its own risks (Daniels 1990b; Light 1992b). Social fairness and actuarial fairness are incompatible, at least in the context of health insurance. The former precludes the latter, and the latter undermines the former.

The United States is unique among nations in having allowed actuarial fairness rather than social fairness to be used for years in medical insurance. Actuarial fairness is widely accepted in private insurance for other kinds of risks, such as fire, theft, and liability coverage, and it requires that people pay insurance premiums that reflect their actual risks. For example, if we owned a wood rather than stone house, or a house more distant from a fire station or fire hydrant, then the greater risks of fire damage would be reflected in our higher insurance premiums. Similarly, a driver with a series of moving violations or record of previous accidents is at higher risk of future accidents and pays a higher premium in most states for automobile insurance.

The intuitive idea behind actuarial fairness in nonmedical insurance contexts is that it is unfair to make people who are at low risk cross-subsidize the security bought by people at high risk when they purchase insurance. In these nonmedical cases, many of the risks we face are the results of other choices we make, for example, what kind of house we buy and where it is located, or how we drive. If we make "safer" choices in houses and driving styles, then it seems only fair that we are entitled to benefit from the savings in premiums that would result if our premiums were risk rated.

Consider now the analogy of this intuitive idea to the case of health risks. The claim would have to be that if people are at lower health risks, then they are entitled to benefit from that trait: it is an asset that is worth something in the insurance market. If the claim were restricted to health risks that are affected by lifestyle choices, then there is some plausibility to it, and we return to that specific subset of health risks later in this discussion of benchmark 4. But most health risks are not affected by choices, and others are only somewhat so and in ways of which we are not aware.

Is there a general rational to support the view that we are entitled to the economic benefits that derive from being at lower risk, even where lifestyle choice is not an issue? One possibility is the general claim that every individual trait, including our levels of health risks, is an asset or resource that we should be entitled to exchange for whatever benefit we can derive. We do not and should not, however, believe this general claim. Skin color is a trait that has market value in some social contexts—whites are paid more than blacks in our society for comparable work. But we are right to think that no one is entitled to benefit in these ways from this kind of individual trait, and we are right to try to prohibit these effects. Both the equal opportunity principle and the European appeal to a social solidarity principle give reasons for rejecting the idea that variation in health risks is an individual "asset" from which each of us is entitled to benefit. That is, both principles reject this rationale for actuarial fairness. So we have good reason not to carry actuarial fairness over from other insurance contexts to health care.

Even in nonmedical insurance contexts, actuarial fairness is not acknowledged as a fundamental principle of fairness. For example, because we think it is important to protect ourselves against uninsured drivers, many states will set insurance rates that partly subsidize high-risk drivers—charging them less than actuarially fair rates—so that the "public good" of having all drivers insured can be maintained. Similarly, insurers have been prohibited from using such techniques as "red-lining"—drawing a red line around a geographical area that contains a substantial minority population—and refusing to issue homeowners or other property protection insurance, even if the red line is a rough indicator of greater insurance risks. We are thus quite willing to override actuarial fairness in any insurance context for reasons of both social policy and distributive justice.

Another reason to think actuarial fairness is not a basic principle of fairness comes from the fact that insurers are motivated to rate premiums by risk largely because of competitive market pressures. If people know they are at lower than average risk, they may seek cheaper premiums. Those who know they are at greater than average risk will be highly motivated to seek insurance. This is called "adverse selection" or "anti-selection," meaning that the people most expensive to insure will tend to flock to insurance pools, threatening the economic stability of insurers. There are two ways to protect against adverse selection: through standard underwriting practices and through making the insurance compulsory. In the absence of mandatory insurance, insurers say that private insurance providers must be able to protect themselves against adverse selection through medical underwriting.

Carrying the concept of actuarial fairness over into health care insurance has dire effects. In the extreme, it undermines the idea of insurance for those most in need. One percent of the population is so sick it consumes 30 percent of medical expenditures, and the sickest 5 percent consume 58 percent (Berk and Monheit 1992). If we could predict who they are, actuarial fairness would call for each of these sick people to pay tens of thousands of dollars in annual premiums or out-of-pocket expenses for uncovered or partially covered services. As insurers in the United States have refined their techniques of risk rating and risk exclusion, they have caused millions of people to lose insurance. They have made millions of others fear job loss or job change. Excluding those at high risk from medical insurance clearly violates our obligations to meet their needs, even if many of the uninsured eventually have their health care needs met one way or another. There is considerable evidence that their needs are not met as well, that they postpone treatment till they are sicker and more costly to treat, and that their mortality and morbidity is increased by the lack of insurance (Hadley, Steinberg, and Feder 1991; Franks, Clancy, and Gold 1993; Stoddard, Peter, and Newacheck 1994).

One reason insurance in the United States often includes "back-end" surcharges on the sick, such as co-payments and deductibles, derives from market-based cost-containment strategies and not insurance underwriting concerns. The United States is unique among nations in believing that higher co-payments are an effective way to contain costs. Such charges may minimize or postpone first visits for nonurgent problems, but this may mean that early detection is also reduced and preventive services are certainly decreased. Significant costs are not saved, because anyone seriously ill is in no position to forego treatment, to shop around, or to assess the merits of costly services. None of the countries that have held their expenditures to a level percent of GNP since the late 1970s has used co-payments as a significant mechanism for cost containment. They correctly regard it not only as ineffective but as a way to shift costs to the sick and thus to undermine equitable financing.

While many people conclude that social fairness and community rating are the right principles, they make an exception for self-induced risks. The exception has some plausibility, as we suggested earlier. It is one thing, for example, to be obliged to protect opportunities through medical assistance when people are ill through no fault of their own. It is quite another to have to bear the burden of deliberate choices others make to engage in risky behaviors. Even if we think we should not paternalistically restrict the lifestyle choices competent people make, by coercing them to behave in ways we think is in their interest, it is still only fair that we should not have to pay the extra costs of their free choices. (If people were not competent to make risky lifestyle choices, we might be justified in stopping them paternalistically; but if they are competent, they should be responsible for the full costs of their choices—or so the argument goes.)

The case for holding people responsible for their choices is usually made against smokers because the consequences of smoking are well-established and costly. But smoking has a strong addictive (i.e., involuntary) element to it. Since most smokers begin their addiction while they are adolescents, while they are particularly vulnerable to various kinds of peer pressures and cultural influences, including special advertising campaigns aimed at them, it may not be the best example of "free and informed" choices for which we should hold people financially responsible (Wikler 1978; World Bank 1993). Skiing, tennis, or running represent truer forms of self-induced risks and would be better, purer cases than smoking. Should there be an orthopedic surcharge for skiers and runners, especially since they recover only to start in again? If one believes in risk rating self-induced risks, the case for a sports medical tax or surcharge is stronger than for a surcharge for smokers. Such a surcharge ignores, however, the fact that many self-induced risks are considered desirable for other reasons, as smoking was for decades.

Even if differential rates or coverages reflecting self-induced health risks were desired, calculating them fairly poses great problems. How would the relative risks of different sports or occupations be fairly calculated? People's natural talents and genetic risks sometimes play a role and make fair risk rating even more difficult. In order to document just what risk-taking behaviors people are doing, an elaborate system of risk monitoring would be needed, a kind of medical police state. *Not* to develop such a system would be still worse—actuarial "fairness" done unfairly.

The principle of community rating means that society should not address the risks of behavior, work, and environment by reducing access to needed health care but by dealing with them directly. Restrictions on advertising cigarettes or taxing them directly are much more fair (and apparently more effective) than discouraging them through health insurance. A tax on the resources used in the behavior (tobacco, alcohol, ski equipment) is closer to the choices made in the behavior than a punitive step such as a surcharge on medical insurance or a denial of coverage. If the desirability of offsetting the extra health care costs induced by smoking, alcohol, or skiing were strong enough, the revenues from these taxes could then be dedicated to meeting health needs without creating special obstacles to access to care.

One further objection to benchmark 4 remains, the paradox we noted earlier. In a community-rated, premium-based system, the well poor will to some extent subsidize the costs of the ill rich, undercutting the principle of fairness reflected in benchmark 5, that people should pay according to their ability to pay. The apparent conflict or paradox disappears once we note that a system can be community rated without being progressively financed, and we are concerned with community rating in a premium-based system only once we have abandoned the goal of securing as progressive a system of financing as possible. In that case, it is still fair to insist that the sick not be made to bear an extra financial burden. It is better to respect one principle of fairness than none, though it is better yet to respect both.

Benchmark 5: Equitable Financing—By Ability to Pay

In our discussion of benchmark 4, we have already touched on part of the justification for benchmark 5. We concentrate here on the rationale for making the system of financing reflect the ability to pay. First a comment on ability to pay.

The ability to pay is not directly proportional to income, because poorer people need disproportionately more of their low incomes just to pay for basic living expenses than do less poor or affluent people. As figure 3-1 shows, if one takes the average gross income in 1993 for each quintile of American households and subtracts their average taxes plus a modest amount (which the second lowest fifth spends) for food, housing, clothing, and transportation, one discovers that the lowest fifth of the nation has no money left over for medical bills, health insurance premiums, movie going, or any other expenses. The second lowest fifth has a meager sum left over ($2796 in 1993) for everything else except the four essentials, and it is not until one reaches the middle fifth that households have enough left over ($12,041) to pay for medical bills or health insurance. Even then, this assumes that the middle fifth spends no more for housing, food, clothing, or transporation than the lower working class. Of course, they do spend more, so the amount they have left over is actually smaller.

Whether the money for the health care system is gathered through taxes, premiums, or related means, it should be based on ability to pay. Tax rates, for example, can readily reflect ability to pay by adjusting the rate to income levels. Even a premium-based system can reflect ability to pay, at least to some extent, if there are appropriate subsidies for premiums, though subsidies would have to reach well into middle-income levels.

Scoring of this benchmark therefore centers on assessing the combined burden of premiums, payroll taxes, income taxes, tax deductions or credits, subsidies, and back-end, out-of-pocket expenses against a measure of people's ability to pay. In the United States, employers have been paying all or most of the health insurance premiums for years, with minimal out-of-pocket expenses until the 1980s. These payments, however, come largely out of wages and are therefore quite regressive. If an employer, for example, is paying on average $4000 for health benefits (or vacation days or other fringe benefits) per employee, that benefit consumes four times the percentage of income for a worker earning $25,000 a year than for a manager earning $100,000 a year. Making health benefits tax deductible causes

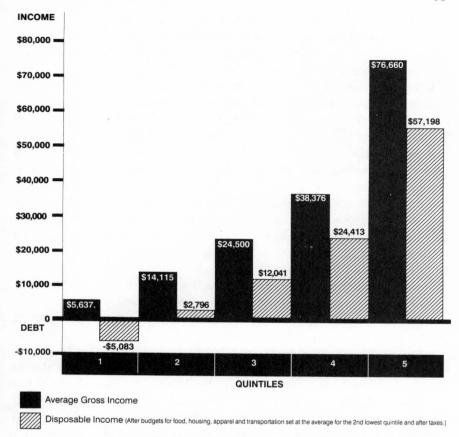

Figure 3–1 Income available for health premiums (by quintiles) 1990.

them to be even more regressive. This is one reason why corporate executives like the current, highly inequitable system of employer-based premiums. They pay a tiny percent of their salary, and the company's premiums produce a huge tax deduction.

Philosophically, theories of justice provide general support for benchmark 5. To illustrate, Rawls' (1971) "justice as fairness" include a principle that constrains allowable inequalities in society in a significant way. Rawls' difference principle says that inequalities permitted by the basic social structure must work to make those who are worst off as well off as possible. This would imply significant transfers of social goods from the best-off members of society to those who are worst off. The principle is compatible with a progressive tax structure, but it does not imply it. How progressive the tax structure should be to satisfy the principle remains an empirical matter.

Similarly, utilitarian theory is compatible with a progressive tax structure but does not directly imply it. A utilitarian would argue that each dollar has a "decreasing marginal utility," so that a dollar will produce less value in terms of the desires it satisfies for someone in the upper income quintile than for someone in the next lower quintile and so on. In theory, we satisfy our most important desires and preferences with our first dollars, leaving later dollars to satisfy less important ones. So an extra dollar to someone with many dollars will be used to satisfy less important preferences, and so produce less satisfaction or welfare, than an extra dollar spent by someone whose more important preferences remain unsatisfied because she is poorer. Although this is in general true, the utilitarian would qualify this rationale for financing by ability to pay by noting that investment, and thus productivity, is negatively affected by steeply progressive tax structures. Just how much a tax structure should reflect ability to pay remains an empirical issue for the utilitarian as well.

We get only general support for the idea of progressivity from these theoretical sources. Our benchmark does not require a precise formula for how charges should be matched to ability to pay. Clearly, premiums reflect ability to pay less well than flat-rate taxes, such as payroll taxes, and payroll taxes reflect ability to pay less well than the federal income tax. We demand no precision beyond this in applying the criterion.

It might be reassuring, however, to find some support for the idea of progressive financing in the values of the American public. The scene is confusing. Our federal income tax was much more steeply progressive through the middle of this century than it became as a result of several recent tax reforms, notably the reform of 1983. In supporting that reform, which retained some progressive tax structure, it was argued that the steep rates of the original code were deceptive because many tax loopholes existed. "Fairness," it was argued, permitted a less progressive rate structure if loopholes were eliminated. That tax reform contributed to the massive transfer in income and wealth from the poor and lower-income groups to the rich during the 1980s, a trend that continues today.

Proponents of a "flat tax" do not argue that progressive financing is unfair but that it is "complex" and that Americans would welcome "simplicity" in tax filing. (Fairness is raised as an issue by opponents of the flat tax, not proponents.) Even the flat-tax proposals are somewhat progressive in that they have high cut-offs for exemption from the tax, but they are clearly regressive above that cut-off. At the state level, support for progressivity varies considerably: some states have only sales taxes, others have income taxes with flat rates, others have more progressive structures.

In short, progressive financing is hardly an un-American, alien idea, for it is embodied in various ways and to varying degrees in our tax structures.

In an antitax, antigovernment climate, however, the appeal to ability to pay is weaker.

Benchmark 6: Value for Money—Clinical Efficacy

We group benchmarks 6 and 7 under the heading "value for money." Benchmark 6 is concerned with the ways in which the use of health care services produces value for money. Benchmark 7 is concerned with other organizational features of the health care system and their impact on obtaining value for money. The British term "value for money" is better than the standard American usage, "efficiency," as Alain Enthoven (1993) acknowledges, because it encompasses several kinds of problems: avoidable duplication, services with little or no benefit, excessive markups and profits, poor organization that wastes money, costly power structures, overprofessionalized services, as well as old-fashioned inefficiencies. The concept of inefficiency comes from industrial production, and sometimes it is pertinent to health care services; but often the so-called inefficiencies are embedded in the professional norms and organization of work (Light 1991b). Value for money is the common denominator for all of these, and the "value" that counts is health status and functioning.

The relationship between value for money and fairness has already been emphasized. Fairness is at issue when health care dollars are spent in ways that do not produce health benefits. Those wasted resources will leave some people with unmet medical needs, or they may force us to spend money from elsewhere in our social budgets, leaving others with unmet educational or housing needs. In short, fairness is at issue in assessing how realistically and fully a proposed reform includes ways to increase value for money. Still, there is a priority here: value for money becomes a matter of fairness because we have obligations to meet peoples' health care needs. We should not make universal coverage or comprehensive benefits, the focus of benchmarks 1 through 3, themselves contingent on achieving more value for money. That would be transposing the priorities.

In both benchmarks 6 and 7, the specific criteria used to measure value for money derive their force from empirical assumptions about how to get value for money, not from assumptions about fairness. In referring to these as assumptions we do not mean they are unsupported. We use the term because we want to signal the importance of them as starting points in an argument about fairness. We believe there is in fact good evidence and theoretical support for these assumptions, which are widely shared. Nevertheless, their application in some cases might produce disagreements, and our purpose throughout this book is to help locate the sources of disagreement so that they can be better understood and resolved.

Benchmark 6 focuses on clinical value. Its scoring centers on the degree to which a proposal sets up a system for minimizing risk factors and the incidence of illness and accidents and then for treating them cost effectively once they occur. We make four key assumptions, each underlying a criterion for this benchmark. The first assumption is that any health reform must retain a strong emphasis on public health and prevention. We are not mindlessly echoing the falsehood that prevention is always cheaper than cure (see Russell 1986, 1994), but we are assuming that it is usually better to prevent an illness or accident than to have to treat it and that it is often cost effective to do so. This assumption is reflected in the criterion calling for reform proposals to emphasize public health and preventive measures.

Despite preventive efforts, illness and trauma will occur and must be treated as effectively as possible within reasonable resource limitations. Our second key assumption about how to achieve value for money is that a reformed system must emphasize primary care. A strong primary-care system can treat 80 to 90 percent of all health problems and is needed to coordinate specialty care (Starfield 1993). Such primary-care systems are prominent in Europe and Canada and contribute significantly to the greater value for money achieved in those systems compared to the United States. Managed care systems that have evolved in the United States have adapted this primary-care foundation to conditions in this country, carefully selecting a layer of primary-care providers who act as a filter before specialists are called in. Primary-care providers should be trained to emphasize preventive measures and to educate patients about lifestyle choices and the self-management of their risks.

A third assumption is that a good plan will promote a more extensive knowledge base than we now have about what interventions work effectively. Many studies have documented wide practice variations in the United States. Medical uncertainty contributes significantly to this variation, and in the context of uncertainty, it becomes easy for practitioners to believe that they should use whatever they have available. Studies have shown that supply, not need or effectiveness, is a key determinant of utilization. A better knowledge base about outcomes and more extensive development of clinical guidelines would reduce this effect.

A fourth assumption is that a good plan will promote ways to minimize both over- and underutilization and that systems should aim to develop ways to avoid both extremes. Carefully thought out reimbursement structures and incentives play an important role in utilization decisions, but these must intend to draw on clinical knowledge, not to introduce extraneous economic incentives. There is considerable concern, for example, that some managed care systems are giving physicians too direct an incentive to make money by undertreating patients. Such incentives reduce value for money and erode professional integrity over time.

Table 3-1. The Cochrane Test for Health Care Systems

1. Focus on what is preventable and prevent it.
2. Focus on diagnosis and what is treatable, not for its own sake.
3. Consider any treatment that is effective.
4. Reduce or eliminate less effective treatments, and make more effective ones available to all.
5. Intervene at the most cost-effective times.
6. Treat at the most cost-effective places.

Many of the points we have made are summarized by the Cochrane Test for effective and efficient health care systems in table 3-1 (Light 1991a).

Benchmark 7: Value for Money—Financial Efficiency

Besides clinical efficacy, a good system will maximize financial efficiency. By this is meant minimizing layers of bureaucracy, installing efficient management systems, exercising financial discipline, minimizing cost shifting, bargaining hard for maximum value in contracts, and preventing fraud and abuse. The four criteria we use for this benchmark draw on a wide array of empirical studies about organizational practices. We emphasize here, as in the previous benchmark, the importance of these empirical assumptions, or starting points.

Before commenting on these assumptions, we note one point that often puzzles people familiar with European health care systems and many domestic critics of the U.S. system, the growth of entrepreneurialism in our system. From the perspective of many people, profits in health care are another troubling source of reduced value. Few other national systems allow profits to be made by directly treating the sick (although in many, individual practitioners are paid on a fee-for-service basis). For-profit health care corporations did not become a significant factor anywhere until the 1970s and even then, almost entirely in the United States (Light 1986).

The frequent assertion that for-profit delivery systems are more efficient has not been supported by comparative research on the subject and appears to be self-serving. Likewise, forms of competition, including managed competition, have not yet been found to reduce overall expenditures after taking into account cost shifting and favorable selection (Congressional Budget Office 1993, 1992; U.S. Government Accounting Office 1993; World Bank 1993; Rice, Brown, and Wyn 1993; Aaron and Schwartz 1993). None of the nations that have halted spiraling costs since the 1970s and held expenditures to a nearly level percent of GNP has used managed competition. The one nation that has transformed its entire delivery system into a form of managed competition, the British National Health Service, has raised expenditures and created new forms of managerial inefficiency. The assertion that competitive systems are organizationally more innovative is also not well supported; significant innovations over the past twenty years have been developed by a small minority of both nonprofit and for-profit delivery systems, while most systems in competitive markets conform to the customs and fashions of the day. Profits in the development and manufacturing of new medical technologies, equipment, and drugs are another matter. They seemed to have spurred important innovations, although most new products in a decade's time add minor features that do not improve clinical diagnosis or treatment or reduce costs.

Despite our concerns about the growth of a for-profit sector in the U.S. system, we have not reflected these concerns in the criteria used in benchmark 7. Instead, we have made four assumptions about how organizational features of a system can increase value for money, and developed criteria that reflect them. (Again, in calling these "assumptions," we intend to focus attention on them as starting points for an analysis of fairness. We chose them because we think they are well-supported assumptions.) No claims about fairness play a role in the rationale for these assumptions; fairness enters in, as in the previous benchmark, because getting less value for money spent is unfair to patients whose health needs are not met and to others whose nonmedical needs are not met when health care budgets are bloated by waste.

Our first assumption is that minimizing administrative overhead will produce more value for money. Administrative overhead takes many forms. Having multiple insurers often means that the mechanisms for claim processing must be duplicated by each insurer, losing important economies of scale. Many insurers rely on highly intrusive case-by-case utilization review, as opposed to "profiling" practice patterns and reviewing outliers. Together, these factors mean that the U.S. system spends a much larger proportion of its health budget on administration than the systems in Europe and Canada. Within the United States, Medicare is administratively far more efficient than the private insurance sector.

Our second assumption is that tough bargaining for rates for services with hospitals, pharmaceutical companies, and clinicians will reduce costs. In some countries, this effect is achieved because of the size of the bargainer: the whole Canadian province, for example, negotiates a budget for reimbursements to physicians, and then the medical associations representing different physicians negotiate a reimbursement structure among themselves that fits within the budget. In the United States, the emergence of large managed care systems in some areas has led to extensive discounting of rates by both hospitals and physicians. Whether true savings result, however, depends on whether or not discounts are followed by cost shifting, so that either subscribers or other insurers pay more.

Value for money then requires a third assumption, that a system or proposal that reduces cost shifting will be more capable of achieving value for money. Cost shifting between private and public sectors must be avoided. Medicare cannot be expected, for example, to make up for reduced hospital revenues that result from discounting services to HMOs. Nor can cost shifting from one part of the private sector to another be allowed to take place. A proposal that pays little attention to the dangers of cost shifting will thus not be as fair, according to this criterion, as one that does.

Finally, we assume that more attention to fraud and abuse within the health care sector would produce more value for money. Good proposals must provide mechanisms and sanctions for these activities.

Each of our assumptions supports one of the four criteria we adopt for scoring this benchmark.

Benchmark 8: Public Accountability

In any health care system, decisions about how to allocate funds and how much money to spend on what types of treatments and services are being made all the time. However, most of these decisions are being done by insurers, employers, benefits administrators, and managed care officers behind closed doors. Policies are cancelled or changed; procedures are denied; providers are dropped with little or no accountability. This situation amounts to managerial elitism, even when managers try to make conscientious decisions (Boren 1994; Peters and Rogers 1994). A public affected by decisions made in this way will react with suspicion. People are likely to conclude, in the absence of any evidence to the contrary, that insurers are making decisions only with "the bottom line" in mind, not patient welfare. They will seek fairness in the courts since they do not sense it in the decisions made about them.

The degree to which a health care system uses democratically developed, unambiguous criteria to make such decisions is an important measure of its fairness. Public accountability in the form of open, democratic processes is a fundamental requirement of justice because people must understand what principles and reasoning are used in choices that affect their basic well-being. This principle applies equally to procedures for handling grievances, an important vehicle for patients and families to voice their concerns in a large complex system. Together, public accountability in decision making and in grievance procedures provides "due process" for patients affected by the public or private bureaucracies we call medical insurance.

Our emphasis on publicly accountable, democratic processes and the explicit provision of reasons for a policy runs counter to one line of thinking (Calabresi and Bobbitt 1978). Hard decisions that often involve limiting life-extending services are sometimes referred to as "tragic choices." Making tragic choices clear and public may call into question fundamental social values, such as the sanctity of life. Some have argued that there is a high social cost to challenging or limiting such values in a public way. It is better, they suggest, to decentralize and even disguise such decisions. Only then can we get reasonable outcomes without paying the full social cost of publicly questioning and limiting important social values. We believe, however, that the requirements of justice for public accountability outweigh these considerations.

Our assumption underlying this benchmark is that fairness requires public disclosure and a trust in the capabilities of people to reason about fairness through democratic processes, despite the risks that arise when we challenge traditional values directly. There is simply no alternative to public accountability because there is no group of managers or professionals who can be relied on to act in ways that are fair to everyone, given their own interests, without having to justify their actions to those affected by their decisions. In this case the price of securing fairness over time is the discomfort of having to discuss and disagree about important issues of value publicly. Some insist this process is a valuable exercise and not a sacrifice. In any case, it is a price that has to be paid, for the cost of not doing so is even greater.

Benchmark 8 is assessed by reference to four criteria. Health care systems have profound effects on the opportunities open to us and quality of our lives, but we are often in the dark about just how well they are working to secure those benefits. One aspect of public accountability is to undertake careful, scientific assessments of the performance of the system as a whole and its various components. Public reporting of these outcome measures is likely to be perceived as threatening to some interests. For example, hospitals and practitioners have opposed the public reporting of mortality statistics by the Health Care Financing Administration, arguing that they are crude measures open to public misunderstanding. But refinements of this sort of evaluation is an essential mechanism for improving the system and relying on consumer choices to force such improvements in quality.

A test for this benchmark is how decisions get made for rationing resources or services, and this is captured in our second criterion. Although clinical and administrative waste should be eliminated first, rationing will have to occur. The *successes* of medicine are a major reason. As medicine can do more for more health problems, its techniques identify still more problems.

The general principles of distributive justice, like the principles assuring equal opportunity, do not help that much when it comes to rationing (Daniels 1993), as we noted in chapter 2. For example, although our concept of fairness makes clear that the sickest patients should be given priority, it does not tell us how *much* priority to give them. Nor does it give us specific principles for weighing significant benefits for a few against modest benefits for many. Collective judgment is also needed on the criteria for "needed" and "effective" services (benchmark 3 and 6), and Callahan points out that practically speaking, efficiency (benchmark 7) involves forms of rationing. If we had a clear consensus on appropriate rationing principles, then we might be able to rely on managers or experts to apply them. But in the absence of clear consensus on such principles, we must rely on fair democratic procedures for making such difficult choices (Daniels and Sabin 1995). These choices are not the premise of any particular set of experts.

Another reason why rationing decisions must be made with full public accountability is that compliance with decisions both by patients and practitioners requires that they are convinced that the decisions are fair. In our current system, where the public suspects that decisions are made by insurers solely with profits in mind, patients and practitioners are unmotivated to comply with even reasonable restrictions. For example, patients threatening litigation can successfully demand unproven technologies, such as autologous bone marrow transplants for breast cancer (see Daniels and Sabin 1995). If decisions restricting access to such therapies were made by fair procedures, in which the rationale was open to scrutiny, criticism, and reasonable appeal, public acceptance of restrictions would become more likely.

Disputes about treatments often arise within provider organizations. The disputes may be between patients and their physicians or between practitioners and the insurer. Our third criterion requires that health care systems provide adequate grievance procedures and mechanisms for dispute resolution at all levels. This criterion applies both to public and private insurers.

The fourth criterion calls for adequate steps to be taken to protect patient privacy and confidentiality, a widely acknowledged issue of fairness in health care systems. Evolving health care systems and technologies for information storage and management expose patients to new forms of violations of privacy. Yet these new systems and technologies are necessary to assure value for money within the system and improved quality of diagnosis and care. Properly designed safeguards can protect privacy and still allow the gains that new systems and technologies promise.

Benchmark 9: Comparability

Benchmark 9 asks that we put health care on a level playing field with other important social goods. Specifically, it asks that all funds expended for health care should be explicitly gathered into a budget so that they can be weighed against other social needs, such as police protection and education. Since global health budgets were not a feature of the recent public debate about health care reform—although they are central to the health care systems of other countries—it needs some introduction and explanation.

We have argued that health care is a good of special moral importance because of its impact on opportunities, but we have also insisted that it is not the only important social good. Education, job training, and job creation, for example, also contribute to the range of opportunities we enjoy. A fair society must also protect fundamental liberties, and it must provide security of person and property. Through the design of its basic institutions, it must promote a stable, growing economy and invest in the science and technology needed for those goals. At the family and individual level, millions of working people have felt the clash between what they spend on health care and their other goals in life. The prospects of real growth in their disposable income have diminished or been lost because of the rapid growth rate in their employee benefits, primarily health care. On both the individual and societal level, then, health care must compete with these other important goods for a reasonable share of social resources.

How should we decide what constitutes a reasonable level of expenditure on health care? Is there some magic number—7 or 10 or 15 percent of gross domestic product—that is "reasonable" or fair? There is no magic number. If we compare rough measures of health care output, such as mortality, infant mortality, and morbidity statistics, then we do see that spending much more as a nation on health care does not necessarily produce better outcomes. U.S. outcomes are measurably worse than those of many countries that spend about half of what we do on health care. More important than the percent of GNP spent on health care is how the system is organized and how the money is spent.

There are basically three strategies for answering the question about how much of GNP to spend on health care. If health care were delivered solely through an unregulated market, individual expenditures that are thought reasonable or necessary by each person would, in the aggregate, determine what society as a whole spent. This strategy is a reasonable and arguably fair way to decide how much society should spend on many things, from bubble gum to computers, although it presupposes that our income distribution is itself a just one. Since we attach some special importance to health care, however, we view it as a good to which we must assure everyone access, including the poor, whether or not we give them insurance. We therefore do not and cannot rely solely on individual expenditures, but we must create some social programs for delivering health care. There are also some "public good" components of health care expenditures, including public health and safety measures, that require public budgets.

The second strategy for deciding how much to spend is to rely on a combination of public and private expenditures to determine a reasonable and fair social outlay. In our version of that strategy, however, public entitlement programs, such as Medicare and Medicaid, are not capped by public budgets, and so cannot be compared in a budget process to other expenditures. In addition, public expenditures end up being the result of millions of individual decisions about health care utilization and expenditure, and these decisions are made against a background of diverse sorts of incentives. In effect, both in public insurance schemes and in private ones, people have no clear way of weighing the importance of health care expenditures against expenditures of other goods. For us, this strategy provides no comparability and is a clear failure.

The third strategy is the one used by nearly every country that has a national health insurance or service system. This strategy is called for by the criterion we employ for benchmark 9. All funds expended for health care should be explicitly gathered into a budget so that they can be weighed against other social needs. In other words, a reform proposal is more fair if it puts health care expenditures on a more equal footing with other social goods than a proposal that does not.

Most other nations place severe limits on how much of their GNP should go to health care. The point at which hijacking is seen as a serious problem, however, varies greatly by political culture. The British restructured their entire health care system in an attempt to keep expenditures below 6 percent of GNP. The Japanese take strong measures at about 7 percent, while the Germans have repeatedly taken action to keep expenditures under 9 percent. American leaders have been talking as if a cost crisis has existed since President Nixon declared one in 1971. Yet only modest or partial measures were taken as health care expenditures rose to 9, then 11, then 13, and now 15 percent of GNP. Gross expenditures are said to be unstoppable before 17 or 18 percent. In a practical sense, this means that Americans have not yet defined a clear limit on the degree to which health care can hijack funds from public programs to meet other needs or from private incomes.

The idea of a global budget is likely to be attacked in several ways in the United States. Some view it as the worst form of government interference with markets. Others complain it will force a comprehensive form of rationing. Others see a threat to research and clinical innovation. For some, it will lead inevitably to the downsizing of health care expenditures and then to reduced services for the poor, since it has only been by unmeasured cross-subsidization that many services have been delivered to the poor in our system.

Each criticism merits a brief response. Global budgets would vastly constrain the growth of markets for health care. They would permit clear priorities to be set between health care and other goods and would force explicit prioritization of expenditures within the health care sector. The experience from other societies is that these steps lead to much greater value for money and to improvements in many measures of health outcomes. This market constraint should be assessed on its merits, not condemned for ideological reasons alone.

To say that global budgets will produce rationing is to ignore the the fact that much rationing goes on in their absence. A global budget would force the weighing of opportunity costs more thoroughly and carefully across all areas of health expenditure. The rationing that results is likely to be more efficient and fairer than what we have now.

Unless budgets build in an allowance for clinical experimentation and other forms of research, they will sharply curtail medical progress. What budgets will force is a social comparison of the value of medical research against other forms of investment in health care services and against other forms of investment in research in other parts of the social budget. Whether this leads to less funding for medical research or not becomes a matter of social choice.

Finally, if other considerations of fairness are met, the needs of the poor will be better met by the system than they are now. Relying on hidden cross-subsidies is an opportunistic strategy—one that is failing in light of market forces now at work—that should not be counted on to produce fairness in health care distribution.

Benchmark 10: Degree of Choice

Benchmark 10 says that a health care reform is fairer than another if it provides for informed choices along four dimensions; choice of primary-care provider, choice of specialist, choice of alternative health care providers, and choice of procedures. The importance of choice to the American public was emphasized in the recent debate about health care reform, most dramatically in the television ads attacking the Clinton proposal. The "Harry and Louise" ad campaign, sponsored by health insurers, attacked the way in which Clinton's "big government" proposals would lead to a loss of choices by the American public. Judging from the effectiveness of that ad campaign, choice is very much on the public's mind, but how is it connected to fairness? Why is it incorporated in this benchmark?

There are two lines of argument that connect issues of choice to concerns about fairness. The first line of argument makes choice a matter of fairness directly. A system is more fair than another, on this view, if the informed, autonomous choices of people are respected in it. A system in which choice is given little importance is thus viewed as more restrictive and even coercive in the limits it imposes on people. This concern about fairness clearly goes beyond the equal opportunity account itself. It has considerable support from various theoretical perspectives and resonates well with American attitudes. Of course, people cannot always have their first choices. Choices sometimes lead to conflict. A fair system cannot simply promise that all choices will be satisfied. This is especially true if satisfying choices in some cases leads to less value for money and less effective care.

Choice is not always in conflict with the search for efficiency and quality, however. A second line of argument for the relationship between choice and fairness appeals indirectly to choice as a way of assuring efficiency and quality. A system that pays little attention to patient satisfaction and the "consumer" aspects of health care delivery may sacrifice important aspects of quality. For example, it might ignore patient time spent in obtaining treatment. Still, many years of research have documented that the criteria by which most patients judge quality differ from the criteria of clinical effectiveness (for example, see Flood, Lorence, Ding, 1993). The best way to assure that patient choice works to support concerns about clinical effectiveness and quality is to provide patients with excellent information about outcomes and performance—of practitioners, managed care systems, and procedures. Our assumption is that choice is an important device for making the health care system better, but it can serve that function only if the system is publicly accountable in the ways required by benchmark 8.

It is important to understand the relationship between choice and other dimensions of fairness, for other dimensions affect the choices open to people. For example, the degree to which people in different insurance schemes are on an equal footing matters considerably. A Medicaid card today is like a credit card limited to a second tier of low-cost and perhaps lower-quality providers. Some of them may be excellent; but the degree and range of choice differ significantly from those for someone who holds a Medicare card or a card to a full service plan. More dramatically, people without insurance have little choice among primary-care providers and often must resort to emergency rooms for care. We leave it to the reader to consider the ways in which improved fairness on benchmarks 1 through 9 will have a positive effect on the choices of most people in the system.

Choice of practitioners and procedures will be reasonably limited by publicly accountable decisions made in light of resource limitations. Not everything people might want to have is part of a fair array of services offered. Some kinds of restrictions on choice will be made, however, primarily for the convenience or profit of the insurer or managed care system, and some of these choices are not justifiable on grounds of fairness. They then constitute unfair restrictions of choice.

We cannot simply say without qualification that more choice is better than less or more is more fair than less. That depends on the operation of other considerations of fairness. But, within reasonable limits, more choice is better than less, and that is what is recognized by this benchmark.

A few comments are in order about the specific criteria for this benchmark. We include a criterion that involves the choice of "alternative" health care providers. Millions of Americans use alternative forms of health care services and believe they benefit from them. We want this dimension of fairness to be constrained, however, by the assessment of efficacy that constrains all services offered in the system. If such alternatives are of demonstrated efficacy, then the fact that they are nonstandard alternatives should not count against them. A similar concern affects choices of procedures. Some restrictions on procedures will be reasonable because they are of unproven efficacy. There will be conflicts in judgment about the efficacy of procedures, however, between providers and patients, on the one hand, and insurers and managed care systems, on the other. Consumer choice does not mean the insurer is always wrong and must concede, but the insurer may be unfairly restrictive here as well. The importance of public accountability in benchmark 8 is aimed at protecting both parties in this dispute by insisting on fairness and accountability in decisions that are likely to be controversial.

Scaling to Assess Reforms

The matrix we have developed can be used for various purposes. In this book, we put the matrix to two different uses. Our primary application (chapters 4 and 5) has the purpose of comparing the fairness of alternative reform proposals for the U.S. health care system. In chapter 6, however, we use it to assess current trends in our system. This application requires a slight change in the interpretation of the scale from its use in earlier chapters. More significant modifications of the matrix could be used to compare the fairness of alternative systems in different countries. Such modifications might add new benchmarks, demote others, or redesign the scale. Just how the scale is constructed should reflect the purpose in using the matrix, just as the shape of a good hammer should depend on its use.

Our primary purpose in this book is to put fairness in the public debate about health care reform. Applying the benchmarks to specific reform proposals, each representing a general type of reform, will thus serve to demonstrate the strengths (and weaknesses) of this tool. The strength we hope is revealed is the way in which it makes obvious the assumptions that underlie judgments about fairness.

To compare the fairness of different health care reform proposals, we must construct a scale for each dimension or benchmark that reflects our purpose and standpoint. In assessing reform proposals, our standpoint is the current system, the status quo. In applying the matrix, the question we ask is whether explicit features of the proposal move us (and in what direction) from the status quo, with reference to the criteria for each benchmark. We suggest a simple scale of −5.0 to 0 to +5.0 with 0.5 intervals, taking the current system (as of summer 1994) or status quo as a zero. This approach allows the entire scale to indicate how the changes introduced by the reform improve or worsen the situation relative to the status quo with reference to the criteria used in each benchmark. Taking zero as the status quo seems a reasonable way to highlight the dimensions of fairness that a given proposal does not address or barely mentions; for no mention or no change will receive a zero. This scale, however, does not measure the overall fairness of the health care system. A zero on this scale might actually be quite unfair relative to some other system. If we were trying to compare alternative systems, e.g, the Canadian, the British, and ours, our scale would have to be modified to reflect our purpose. On the whole the proposals for reforming the American system that we examine in chapters 4 and 5 increase its fairness, but a few features of some plans are noted for making the present system worse.

In chapter 6, we put the benchmarks to a slightly different use. Our key question is whether trends currently at work in the U.S. health care system are making the system fairer or not with respect to each benchmark. For this purpose, we take as our baseline the summer of 1994, roughly marking the failure of efforts at comprehensive governmental reform in the 103rd Congress. Although we still use a scale from −5.0 to 0 to +5.0, there is a subtle change in the meaning of the scores. For example, a zero on a criterion in chapter 4 or 5 means that the reform proposal involves no steps that alter the unreformed system for that criterion. A zero in chapter 6 means that the trends at work in the system do not alter fairness relative to the baseline. As a result a proposal that did not improve coverage relative to the unreformed system received a zero in Chapter 4, but if the trends at work increase the numbers of uninsured, as they seem to be doing, then a negative score might be given in chapter 6 for the same criterion.

All of our decisions about the details of the benchmarks and the scale to be used for them are open to revision. Others may wish to devise a different scale for the benchmarks or alter the details of the criteria for scoring benchmarks. We welcome efforts to make it a better tool.

There are two related objections to our approach that we would like to address here. The first objection is that there is something peculiar about trying to put numbers on moral judgments, including judgments about fairness. We do not say that murder is a "10" and rape only a "7," or that deliberate deception of a friend a "6" and deception of a stranger a "5." So why construct a scale that assigns a numerical value to ten dimensions of fairness? Why pretend to do moral mathematics? The second objection is that our use of numbers is confusing: sometimes they suggest a real comparison of quantities (a cardinal scale), sometimes only a relative or positional ranking (an ordinal or even just a qualitative scale). The objection is that we should not use numbers unless we want them to be taken seriously and think there really is a metric that gives them uniform meaning.

The answer to the first objection is that we do not pretend to be doing moral mathematics. We hope our numbers are not taken more seriously than we intend them or out of the context in which we use them. We intend them primarily to provide a graphic way of representing the fact that some reforms do more than others to improve our system in ways that affect specific aspects of fairness. Although we do not ordinarily assign numbers to violations of moral (or legal) rules, we do think some violations are more serious than others. We do not ordinarily have reason to represent these judgments about seriousness in a systematic way. We do not plot, for example, the moral improvement in our children along the many dimensions that constitute the virtue of showing consideration for others.

If we had special reason for doing so, however, we might well want to plot moral improvement in a quantitative way. If our child exhibited some difficulty in showing consideration for others, we might set up a system of rewards and punishments, attempting to modify her behavior in specific ways. Part of that plan might include awarding so many "stars" or "points" for performing specific tasks that involve more and less complex forms of showing consideration for others. We might even praise the child for having a good day in which twelve points were earned, rather than six. The point is not to teach the child moral mathematics, and this is not the lesson the child draws. The child learns that some behaviors are seen as more seriously wrong than others, and some actions much more praiseworthy than others. These numbers have no meaning outside the context of the plan and its purpose, and not one psychologist, parent, or child gets confused about this fact. The scores simply provide a graspable way of referring to many more specific criteria and the degree to which they have been satisfied.

Our numbers are intended to do no more than the numbers in the child's system of rewards. In reforming a complex health care system, we have reason to analyze the many ways in which changes may affect fairness and to represent the results of that analysis in a way that facilitates comparisons about the relative importance of different outcomes. The numbers are an aid to keeping track of the results of many particular judgments and analyses. They are not more precise than the particular analyses they conveniently represent. Nor do they have any meaning outside the meaning assigned by the scale and criteria used. We are not substituting moral mathematics for moral reasoning.

We can now reply to the second objection, that our numbers are confusing. We seriously considered presenting only qualitative comparisons (see Daniels 1995, chapter 8, where only qualitative charts are used.) We concluded, however, that a matrix scorable by numbers would be more readily graspable than a vast array of peculiar symbols. For the numbers to be helpful rather than confusing—as they are for the child in the behavior modification program—the focus must always be on the underlying criteria that specify the notion of fairness. It must be clear that the numbers are defined only in the context of the criteria and scale we use. Like the child, who must internalize a way of thinking about specific behaviors and ultimately a disposition to show consideration in different ways for others, we must internalize a way of thinking about the impact on fairness of specific features of health care reform.

This warning that the numbers are not real and derive their meaning or reference only from the criteria for our benchmarks must be taken seriously and must be kept in mind even when our own procedure might seem to grasp at the reality of the numbers in specific cases. For example, in benchmark 1, where we are interested in the degree to which a proposed reform closes the insurance gap of 15 percent uninsured, it is natural to think of the point scale we propose as referring to real magnitudes (as a true cardinal scale), and we draw on this natural interpretation in our own scoring. A plan that closes one-third of the gap should get a score half as great as a plan that closes two-thirds of the gap. The situation is quite different, however, when we apply numbers to score the degree to which a plan pays attention to the need for eliminating clinical waste (benchmark 6) or administrative complexity (benchmark 7) or public accountability (benchmark 8) or choice (benchmark 10), where there are no natural magnitudes associated with the criteria. (There might be such a magnitude in the case of clinical efficacy if we could establish exactly how much medical utilization is "unnecessary" or "wasteful" and make accurate estimates of reduction in those numbers by different proposals; we can do neither.)

In short, we are not attempting to create moral mathematics, and we are not pretending our numbers are real or have meaning beyond the way they are specified in the matrix. The goal is to focus our attention graphically on the underlying problem—what aspects of fairness are affected in what ways by specific features of reform proposals. The analogy to the child's behavior modification program is again apt: Our problem is to modify our behavior as policy analysts, as politicians, and as the public. We must think about how fairness is affected by what we do and approve, just as the child must think about how her behavior exhibits consideration for others. The num-

Table 3-2. Benchmarks of Fairness for National Health Care Reform

Benchmark 1:	Universal access—Coverage and Participation
	Mandatory coverage and participation
	Prompt phase-in: Coverage/participation not held hostage to cost control
	Full portability and continuity of coverage
Benchmark 2:	Universal Access—Minimizing Nonfinancial Barriers
	Minimizing maldistributions of personnel, equipment, facilities
	Reform of health professional education
	Minimizing language, cultural, and class barriers
	Minimizing educational and informational barriers
Benchmark 3:	Comprehensive and Uniform Benefits
	Comprehensiveness: All effective and needed services deemed affordable, by all effective and needed providers. No categorical exclusion of services, like mental health or long-term care.
	Reduced tiering and uniform quality
	Benefits not dependent on savings
Benchmark 4:	Equitable Financing—Community-Rated Contributions
	True community-rated premiums
	Minimum ddiscrimination via cash payments
Benchmark 5:	Equitable Financing—By Ability to Pay
	All direct and indirect payments and out-of-pocket expenses scaled to household budget and ability to pay
Benchmark 6:	Value for Money—Clinical Efficacy
	Emphasis on primary care
	Emphasis on public health and prevention
	Systematic assessment of outcomes
	Minimizing overutilization and underutilization
Benchmark 7:	Value for Money—Financial Efficiency
	Minimizing administrative overhead
	Tough contractual bargaining
	Minimize cost shifting
	Anti–fraud and abuse measures
Benchmark 8:	Public Accountability
	Explicit, public, and detailed procedures for evaluating services, with full, public reports
	Explicit democratic procedures for resource allocation
	Fair grievances procedures
	Adequate privacy protection
Benchmark 9:	Comparability
	A health care budget, so it can be compared to other programs
Benchmark 10:	Degree of Consumer Choice
	Choice of primary-care provider
	Choice of specialists
	Choice of other health care providers
	Choice of procedure

bers graphically remind us of crucial differences in what we do and may motivate us to do better.

Summary

We offer the matrix formed by these benchmarks and the criteria for scoring them as a basis for including fairness in the debate about health care reform. It provides a framework that can be used by policy experts, state legislators, and representatives, as well as the public, to assess the relative fairness of alternate proposals for universal health care. By making explicit the moral and empirical assumptions underlying each benchmark and each criterion, we hope to improve debate about fairness. Being straightforward allows people to focus on the source of their agreements and disagreements and to see why matters thought unrelated to judgments about fairness really are related to them. Our benchmarks and the criteria for them are summarized in table 3-2.

In the next three chapters we illustrate the use of the matrix in two different tasks. First, we examine carefully four specific reform proposals presented in the 103rd Congress. Our interest is not antiquarian, however, for we select these proposals as examples of more general types of reform proposal we might encounter in a serious effort to reform the system. Second, we use the matrix in a somewhat modified way to make judgments about the market-driven "reorganization without reform" that characterizes the period immediately after the 103rd Congress. We emphasize throughout that we see the tool we are using here as one that must be refined through the practical effort of using it.

4

Using the Benchmarks to Score Insurance Reforms

The benchmarks of fairness and their criteria show what is ethically at stake when important choices are made about the design of reform proposals. Our task now is to show how they can be used in practice to compare the fairness of alternate proposals. We do not intend to use the scores we assign to talk down opponents or seize the moral high ground or end discussion about fairness. Rather, we offer the benchmarks as an analytic tool that can improve debate about fairness by making it more substantive and specific. The question is, How best to illustrate their use?

One easy, clean way would be to use hypothetical reform proposals. Although hypothetical proposals might have allowed us to consider more pure, generic types of reform, they would lack the kinds of detail needed to engage our criteria for scoring the benchmarks. They would also be less real to the reader. They might have allowed us to construct our own ideal reform—the perfect five on our scale—but that is not the purpose of this book. We decided to stay real. Despite the risk of seeming outdated, we chose to evaluate four complete, actual, national-scale proposals from the 103rd Congress. By selecting them carefully, we thought they could represent a wide range of the reform ideas that have dominated American debate for many years, and they would have greater breadth than some interesting state efforts.

The four bills we chose to evaluate can be arrayed on a spectrum running from "free market" to "government" approaches. The Michel bill, "Affordable Health Care Now," represents those policies that emphasize a voluntary, market-oriented approach to coverage and cost containment. There are no global budget or premium caps, but instead a series of reforms to correct problems in the health insurance market and provide subsidies for low-income people. The goal is to allow more people to participate in the private market and to focus the market more sharply on price and quality. This approach does not mandate coverage and does not require employers to pay premiums for health insurance. It organizes the small-group market and allows states to form voluntary purchasing co-operatives for small employers. With some exceptions, it leaves to the market such issues as benefits coverage, degree of cost sharing, and standards of quality. Government participation is minimal, and it is the least expensive to implement. It might be characterized as the "free market" approach, though all markets have some regulation, and private health care markets require a great deal of regulation to avoid people being harmed (Enthoven 1988, 1993). We shall refer to the Michel bill as the *market-based approach.*

The Cooper bill, the "Managed Competition Act," represents a more structured or regulated use of market forces and voluntary participation. For example, it proposed a system of state and regional purchasing pools, required a standard benefits package with an emphasis on free preventive services, replaced Medicaid with a low-income assistance program to allow people to purchase private insurance as well, and took various measures to slow the growth of Medicare expenditures. While this approach also does not set premium caps or global budgets, it goes further in reforming the private insurance market by requiring age-adjusted community rating, renewability, portability, quality standards, and by limiting the use of preexisting condition clauses. These reforms aim to make private health insurance equitable so that competition rewards efficiency and performance more than it does now. This might be called the *lightly managed competition approach.*

The Clinton bill, the "Health Security Act," represents a reform approach that combines guaranteed universal coverage with competition to control costs. Coverage is comprehensive, specified, and includes long-term and community-based care as well as preventive services. This approach regulates and manages competitive markets more thoroughly than the other two, through detailed stipulations to create parity and through oversight bodies, in this case, regional health alliances. Through limited cost sharing, capitated health plans, pure community rating, uniform quality standards, and various incentives, this approach gives purchasers encouragement to reward more cost-effective plans. The Clinton bill also proposed spending reductions in Medicare and Medicaid, and taxes on cigarettes and large corporations to control costs. Many other parts dealt with fuller and better designed coverage for the elderly and the poor. The bill was estimated to cost more than fifteen times as much to implement as the first two bills. Proposals of this kind could be called the *heavily managed competition approach.*

The McDermott/Wellstone bill, the "American Health Security Act," emphasized universal coverage for health care and budgetary cost containment. This approach eliminates private insurance, Medicare, and Medicaid and replaces them with a single, government-sponsored insurance plan financed through taxes. All the money now spent on private insurance gets rechanneled into this plan. In a similar spirit, this approach establishes national standards for coverage and quality. Services are free at the point of delivery; there are no forms of cost sharing (except for long-term care), because it is regarded as regressive, discriminatory, and not very effective at containing costs. Rather, this approach relies on using national and state global budgets together with fee schedules and institutional budgets to hold costs down. This is known as the *single-payer approach,* because all funds get directed to a single payer. It roughly resembles the Canadian health care system.

In using these bills as vehicles for assessing a wide spectrum of health reform proposals in the various states and the nation, we will examine them much more closely. These sketches only summarize some of the characteristic features of each. The benchmarks too are only schematic, which is why we decided that assessing real bills would help to show others how they can use them in assessing other health policies and practices. This process necessarily combines theoretical and empirical considerations, so that if evidence or practices change, they may affect the scores. As we explained in chapter 3, it is important to keep clear in one's mind differences of values from differences of data or empirical assumptions about how the world works. Clarifying these differences, in fact, is a principal benefit of formulating and using the benchmarks, as we illustrated with the debate about whether making universal coverage contingent on saving money first is fair or unfair.

Our scoring procedure began with reading separately the bills and related materials in order to identify which features address which criteria for each of the ten benchmarks. We then discussed in great detail our individual reasons for giving each proposal a score on each criterion. Disputes and questions necessitated further investigation and more conversations until we agreed on the scores. Another team of raters might score the plans differently. What matters most are the *relative differences* between scores for the proposals. By consistently using the same rating team and applying the same criteria in the same manner, we maximized the consistency of the relative scores.

As mentioned in chapter 3, we have taken the status quo to be zero on our scale for each benchmark and we score on a scale of -5.0 to -5.0 the degree to which features of a bill would make the American health care system more or less fair than it was when the bills were being debated in 1994. For example, given that about 38 million people, or around 15 percent of the population, have no health insurance and the number was rising under managed competition (Iglehart 1995b; Hellander et al. 1995), a plan that would leave 10 percent still uninsured would earn only about 1.5 points out of 5.0 on the criterion for universal coverage. Insuring the first 5 percent is much easier than the next 5 percent, or the last 5 percent. The score would also be affected by how inclusive the definition was of people who had a right to health care when sick. As we noted in chapter 2, however, other criteria for benchmarks do not usually correspond to a cardinal scale, as in this case, and our scale is generally not intended to indicate more than a rough ordinal ranking.

While pegging contemporary practices in the middle of the scale, at zero, has certain advantages, it is important to note that Americans live in the most unfair health care system in the industrialized world. No other affluent nation (and few of the less affluent nations) fails to guarantee universal access to medical services regardless of income, ethnicity, age, or health condition (benchmark 1 and 2). No other allows coverage or premiums to vary by risk or health condition (benchmark 3). No other collects funds so that those who earn less must pay proportionately more of their take-home check for health insurance than those who earn more (benchmarks 4 and 5). No other comes close to being as inefficient as the American system, where about 23 percent of people's premiums go to administration, marketing, and profits (benchmark 7). Few other nations make it so difficult as the United States to compare and decide publicly how much to spend on health care versus other social programs (benchmark 8 and 9). Most disturbing today, few comparable nations are limiting patient choice of specialists and treatments as are American managed care systems (benchmark 10). *Thus, any reform proposal that does not score at least a 4.0 on a given benchmark means that Americans would continue to experience less fair health care services than do residents of other industrialized countries.*

The criteria for each benchmark were described in chapter 3. In what follows, we score each criterion and average the scores for each benchmark. We come down hard on vagueness, promises without much to back them up, and a lack of concern for issues of fairness. Or to put it the other way around, our main conclusion is that too many proposals neglect these issues altogether or substitute unclear declarations for seriously thought-out measures.

Benchmark 1: Universal Access—Coverage and Participation

This benchmark is scored on three criteria: (1) mandatory participation and automatic coverage, (2) prompt phase-in, with participation not held hostage to cost control, and (3) full portability and continuity of coverage. Consequently, a perfect score of 5.0 for the benchmark would require a perfect score on all three fronts. Such a reform would cover everyone living in the country in a nondiscriminatory way; assure continuous, portable coverage; and not make universal coverage dependent on savings. For reasons already explained in chapter 3, universal coverage is the best way to control costs and reduce illness.

Mandatory Coverage and Participation

The single-payer approach as represented by the McDermott/Wellstone bill came close to a perfect score for universal coverage and participation. It assured automatic coverage to and participation by everyone legally living in the country, except veterans and American Indians. The more contentious issue concerned illegal residents. In states like Texas and California, they are prevalent and constitute a significant financial burden. Yet they also make a large, if dubious, contribution to the quality of life for most voters as members of the underpaid, shadow labor market that picks crops, prepares food, washes dishes, buses tables, sews clothes, occupies sweatshops, washes cars, gardens, and tends children. They get no health insurance as a fringe benefit, which is part of their exploitation. They also reproduce the basic American pattern of desperately trying to get to America any way they can in order to find a better life for themselves and their loved ones.

Ironically, each previous generation of immigrants looks with disdain on new groups of immigrants. But the essential issue is that they get sick, as do criminals, prostitutes, or any other class of outcasts. In our view, needed and effective health care must be available to all. Therefore, we believe the exclusion of any given class of individuals is unfair. The central problem for Texas, California, or other places burdened with many immigrants is that Medicaid and/or state programs force those areas to pay a great deal. The expense of illegal immigrants or other costly groups should be borne by the nation as a whole. In the American context, we docked this proposal half a point, giving it a 4.5 on the first criterion.

Universal coverage, combined with managed competition to make the delivery of services efficient, is a common approach to reform, and one version was the original Clinton plan. On the matter of universal coverage and participation, it was nearly as strong as the single-payer approach. Coverage, however, was not quite so automatic, because competing insurance plans would probably try to avoid high-risk subscribers through indirect forms of risk rating that would still be possible under rules of community rating (Light 1992b; Stone 1993). Prohibiting such practices would be difficult. In the case of the Clinton bill, illegal residents and prisoners were not included in the program, and any groups excluded weakens a score on benchmark 1 for the reasons discussed above. The Clinton proposal also had an additional structural flaw of risk-aversive competition. For these reasons, we gave the original Clinton proposal a score of 4.0 on benchmark 1.

Some reform proposals use managed competition but with far less management of the market than the Clinton-type approach. Although this difference matters greatly later on, it does not matter much for benchmark 1, because coverage and participation are largely independent of provider competition. It helps to realize that all reform proposals or actual plans have two distinct parts—how the money is collected and how it is allocated (Light 1994b). Almost any combination is possible. For example, one could collect the money through private insurance and then have a single-payer-type fee schedule and hospital budgets. Conversely, one could have a "single-payer" collection through taxes and a competitive market among providers. Thus, market-oriented reforms can score very high on the first five benchmarks if they create a universal, equalized arena in which the competition takes place.

The problem for reform proposals like that of Senator Cooper is that no universal coverage was mandated. It neither required employers to provide coverage nor individuals to buy it. During annual enrollment periods of no less than thirty days, people could enroll in health plans if they wished. Thus the Cooper proposal did little to reduce the number of uninsured, and its design would discourage low-risk people from participating. Subsidies were to be provided, but few details were given about their size and structure. According to the Congressional Budget Office (1994:20), this proposal would have left 24 million people without coverage, or about 9 percent of the population. For its modest reduction of inequities in universal coverage and participation, the Cooper plan received a 1.5 on benchmark 1.

The market-based Michel bill involved little management of competition compared to the Cooper and Clinton bills, but this hands-off approach is a delivery feature and is distinct from how funds are collected. A conservative approach to the market could be combined with several forms of universal coverage. Unfortunately, the Michel bill had nearly the same problems as Cooper. It excluded illegal residents from coverage, and the status of prisoners was unclear. Coverage for eligibles was neither mandatory nor automatic. Given the highly skewed nature of medical costs, a voluntary insurance system tempts people at low risk to forego insurance until they become sick, thereby making universal coverage all but impossible to achieve. At the same time, under this bill, insurers would have been required to take whomever applied. Voluntary health insurance also leads to higher premiums and less coverage for those at risk, and of course people cannot get health insurance unless they can afford the premiums. The inverse coverage law holds that the more people need health insurance, the less coverage they are likely to get and the more they will pay for it (Light 1992b). The Michel plan permitted, but did not require, states to provide subsidies for individuals up to 200 percent of poverty. It allowed states to include other uncovered individuals, such as part-time workers, in the program, but they would have to pay the entire costs themselves. For these reasons, we estimated that this plan would not expand coverage much, and scored it a 0.5. As already mentioned, these low scores for weakly regulated or unregulated approaches to universal health care are not inherent in the approaches themselves.

Prompt Phase-in

The speed and terms of the phase-in of universal coverage constitute the second criterion, because the length of delay for those without insurance and the terms under which they would eventually be included are matters of fairness. If phase-in depends on a board or a legislature deciding something, or specifying how it will happen, such provisions delay implementation and may alter it. If phase-in is contingent on some other provision, like saving money, it may never happen.

Proposals by committees of the 103rd Congress to use "hard triggers" or "soft triggers" would reverse this contingency but cause delay. For example, hard triggers would be "pulled" and impose mandatory universal coverage if voluntary measures have not achieved a specified increase in coverage after a specified period. Soft triggers return the issue to Congress for further consideration and thus delay phase-in indefinitely. Thus, if the Clinton proposal had been modified to include a five-year hard trigger, we would have reduced its score on the phase-in criterion by at least two points. A soft trigger would have been even more unfair to those who did not have guaranteed health insurance. It would not have assured universality within a specified period, leaving those without insurance hostage to the vagaries of the economy and future health care costs and to the future political will of another Congress. Triggers that would not have been pulled if less than 4 or 5 percent of the population were uninsured (some 10 million people) are still worse; they redefine what "universal coverage" means. In matters of fairness, it is vital to remember how inequitably the burden of health costs falls.

In the case of the specific bills we are using to illustrate the book's themes, the McDermott/Wellstone plan got a 4.5 for prompt phase-in with no contingencies. We gave the Clinton bill a 4.0, because it was unclear whether states could delay their participation. The Cooper bill had purchasing cooperatives electing their boards and *then* deciding if they want to expand coverage. It also makes additional coverage subject to savings, although how one decides when the savings are enough is anyone's guess. These provisions received a 2.0. The more voluntary approach of Michel did little more than require employers to offer a range of plans, and therefore received a score of 1.5.

Portability

The last criterion in this benchmark concerns portability—the continuity of coverage for people changing jobs or residences. A plan like the McDermott/Wellstone bill with no portability problems would receive a 5.0. This would mean no waiting periods or contingencies, no gaps or lapses in coverage, and no problems in switching from one plan to another. The Clinton plan made portability contingent on joining a new alliance. Employees of large corporations who left them might also experience some dislocations as they switched to a health alliance, and therefore it was rated a 4.0. An approach like the Cooper bill has several obstacles to complete portability. For example, health care plans could deny enrollment based on resource constraints or preexisting conditions. With respect to preexisting conditions, people without health insurance coverage would be treated differently (i.e., denied coverage up to six months) from people with coverage. Consequently, those people who most need immediate coverage would be the least likely to get it. Forced disenrollment for nonpayment of premiums would have interfered with continuity of care. And the lack of detail in the plan made it difficult to determine portability for people leaving their regions or switching employment. We gave this proposal a 2.0 on portability.

The relation between coverage and payment is a critical one. While benchmark 1 calls for universal coverage and participation, all fair systems in the world do not cut off benefits if payments are delayed or not paid. These payments are almost always fringe benefit contributions or taxes. If there is a problem in payment, such as tax fraud or wage contributions stopping because a person is laid off, it does not affect his or her eligibility for medical care. Even if people are under criminal investigation and become ill, there is no question that they get medical attention.

This widely practiced concept of fairness contrasts with a voluntary system, in which benefits depend on paying premiums. For example, the Michel bill allowed health plans to cancel or deny coverage for nonpayment of premiums, fraud, "noncompliance with requirements," or for the "misuse of a provider network." The bill prohibited waiting periods, but it eliminated preexisting condition exclusions only for pregnant women, newborns, and people with six months or more of continuous coverage. For everyone else, these exclusions were limited to six months. Thus, the Michel bill received a score of 1.5 because it would have improved portability a little but less than the Cooper bill.

Averaging the scores for benchmark 1, we arrive at the following values:

McDermott/Wellstone	4.7
Clinton	4.0
Cooper	1.8
Michel	1.2

Benchmark 2: Universal Access—Minimizing Nonfinancial Barriers

Providing access to services requires eliminating nonfinancial barriers as well as those imposed by inadequate insurance coverage. Any proposed reforms should be scored on the degree to which they (1) minimize maldistributions of personnel, equipment, and facilities, including provisions for underserved areas; (2) reform health professional education, especially to meet the need for primary-care and minority practitioners; (3) minimize language, cultural, and class barriers to access; and (4) minimize educational and informational barriers to treatment. This benchmark comes second, not only because it complements the removal of financial barriers represented by benchmark 1, but also because it provides a strong test of how seriously a given reform addresses the fundamental inequalities embedded in the history, structure, and culture of the health care system.

Minimizing Maldistributions

Maldistributions of personnel, equipment, and facilities are extensive and difficult to rectify. Yet they affect access and create forms of *de facto* rationing. One effort, like the Certificate of Need (CON) program of the 1970s, attempts to control construction and the purchase of large equipment so that underservice and duplication are minimized. Since the CON program did not work well, because boards got captured by hospital executives, even higher marks should go to reforms that address such past failures and attempt to avoid them.

A second, related idea is to have minorities or the medically underserved participate on advisory boards. This too has been tried in the 1970s, with mixed success. However, the weaknesses of past efforts can be overcome. For example, such representatives need a professional staff or else they find themselves relying entirely on information supplied by providers. Lay representatives face providers who are full-time professionals with their own support staff.

A third, and important, way to address maldistributions is to support programs like the National Health Service Corps or to pay providers more for serving disadvantaged people. The British, despite their small budget (one-third as many dollars per person as the United States), pay their physicians up to 70 percent extra to treat individuals from deprived neighborhoods. Their deprivation scale takes into account the greater illness in these neighborhoods and the greater difficulty in treating patients there. At a macro level, maldistributions can be rectified by allocating proportionately more resources to states with underserved areas, though one must be careful that the middle-class areas of those states do not end up with more than their fair share, as happened with the Hill-Burton program after World War II.

As an example of scoring, the single-payer approach represented here by McDermott/Wellstone did almost all three of these and therefore warranted a score of 5.0. Its features offered both long-term and short-term solutions to current inequities, and most would have been mandatory.

The Clinton bill also devoted considerable attention to current inequities in maldistribution. It greatly increased funding for the National Health Service Corps and for the training of primary-care providers. It made loans available to construct more facilities for mental health and substance abuse, as well as to upgrade facilities to accommodate the comprehensive benefit package. It increased financial incentives for physicians to locate in underserved areas. It required health plans to include essential community providers in their area who wanted to join, and the bill offered financial incentives to enroll disadvantaged populations. The bill contained anti-discrimination provisions to protect both consumers and providers in underserved areas. This is a strong package that shows impressive concern for redressing current maldistributions, and it earned a 4.5. Only the maldistribution of equipment is not adequately addressed.

The Cooper bill consisted entirely of options, not mandates. They would have taken a long time, if ever, to work. For example, the bill encouraged but did not require health plans to locate in underserved areas. Most major areas of concern, like planning for the redistribution of equipment and facilities, were not adequately addressed. For example, purchasing cooperatives would supposedly receive increased compensation for serving underserved areas, but states did not have to fund these increases. All funding was either unspecified or seemed inadequate. The Cooper proposal barely improved any maldistribution and therefore received a 0.5.

The Michel bill was a paradox of heightened sensitivity to the problems of maldistribution together with tepid action. It would have helped community and migrant health centers, but with only $300 million a year. It took up the plight of small rural hospitals with heavy loads of Medicare patients by offering $70 million for one year only. It would have established an Office of Emergency Medical Services to improve rural emergency services, and made grants available to begin air transport systems. It proposed federal grants for up to seven states to improve telecommunications between rural and urban facilities. It made federal grants available to coordinate outpatient primary-care services in underserved areas. To address the problem of physician shortage areas, the bill asked the Secretary of Health and Human Services to make recommendations about how to encourage physicians to volunteer. This is the kind of proposal that earns almost no points because it is vague, voluntary, and indirect.

The bill left unaddressed many key problems concerning the distribution of services and made only minor funding available, largely for emergency services in rural areas and little else. No provision was made in the bill to review the purchase, lease, or construction of facilities or equipment, so their maldistribution would continue. We gave the bill a score of 0.5 on this criterion.

The high scores of McDermott/Wellstone and Clinton and the low scores of Cooper and Michel are not inherent in their overall approaches. One could imagine a single-payer plan that did nothing to redress past maldistributions but instead locked them in. This can be found in some national health plans of developing countries, where the elites retain the inequities of the past as they universalize health care. Conversely, one could imagine a highly market-oriented, private system that started by eliminating past maldistributions so that competition began level. If anything, equality is more vital to a competitive approach, and thus the low scores for the competitive reforms are particularly disappointing.

Reform of Health Professional Education

The second criterion involves reform of health professional education. This is harder to score, because any change in education takes a long time to affect services, and there can be many a slip between lip and cup. The McDermott/Wellstone bill illustrates as well as any how far a proposal can go in an area characterized by long lags and indirect effects. It required each state to establish a separate account for health professional educational expenditures and to distribute funds so that more primary-care practitioners and fewer specialists would be trained. The bill mandated the training of more midlevel practitioners and nonprofessional outreach workers. It established an Advisory Committee on Health Professional Education and doubled funding for health professional education.

These are important measures, but the advisory committee lacked the power to do much against the powerful vested interests of academic medicine. The bill failed to address the relatively small number of minorities in medical education. The bill was also vague about how its redistribution of funding would work. Overall, we gave it a 4.0 on this criterion.

The Clinton proposal also contained many programs and features to promote the training of primary-care physicians, nurses, and other personnel. Most of the money would come from a 1.5-percent assessment on premiums to health alliances and 1 percent on premiums to corporate alliances. Why they should contribute less was unclear. Also, the bill did little to increase disadvantaged minorities going into medicine. We decided it warranted a 4.0 on this criterion.

The Cooper proposal had many good initiatives in professional education. It proposed a national commission to allocate entry positions among medical residency training programs to help correct geographic maldistributions. It would have funded medical residency and physician retraining programs for primary care from a 1-percent tax on gross premiums. It expanded scholarship and loan-repayment programs under the National Health Service Corps and extended the training of various types of allied health professionals. However, most of these measures were voluntary and long-range; so we scored it a 4.0.

The Michel bill contained no educational reforms and received a score of zero on this criterion for no change from the status quo.

Minimizing Language, Culture, and Class Barriers

The third criterion concerns linguistic, cultural, and class barriers. Many field studies over the past forty years have documented the power of such barriers to prevent treatment and cause misunderstanding. Yet none of the four bills we are assessing here addressed them much, and many state reforms do little to correct these barriers. This reflects an insensitivity to the problems described, for example, in *Mama Might Be Better Off Dead* (Abraham 1993) and LuAnn Aday's important analysis *At Risk in America* (1992).

The two most market-oriented bills, Michel's and Cooper's, did nothing to help people who speak English with difficulty, have different concepts about what is making them sick, or live in deprived circumstances that significantly affect their ability to get help or to carry out a treatment plan. By contrast, in the market-oriented reforms of Mrs. Thatcher, the health service offers call-up translation (of language and culture) services for nineteen different languages and dialects in London. The two American bills received a zero.

The Clinton bill contained some efforts. States could provide for outreach, transportation, interpretation, and other services to ensure access, but these are voluntary. Some funding is provided for mental health, substance abuse, and school-based health programs. The bill mainstreamed Medicaid into the private sector. However, child care and other kinds of home and work-related barriers to care were not addressed. We believe these provisions warranted a score of 3.0.

The McDermott/Wellstone proposal allowed payments to community-based primary-care health facilities to reflect the costs of transportation and translation. The bill also abolished Medicaid and mainstreamed the poor. However, cultural barriers, child care, and other kinds of home and work-related barriers were not discussed, and the bill failed to provide for the education needed to overcome them. What measures exist are voluntary. For these reasons, McDermott/Wellstone receives a score of 2.0.

Minimizing Educational and Information Barriers

This criterion of fairness is also vital to effective health care markets, and the two market-oriented bills did much better here than on cultural and class barriers. The Cooper bill required that purchasing cooperatives distribute information about prices, health outcomes, and enrollee satisfaction of alternative plans prior to each annual enrollment period. It authorized a national commission to collect, analyze, and widely distribute financial and clinical information, including the relative performance of each purchasing cooperatives.

These provisions would have made the current system significantly more fair, though they could be stronger. For example, there were no measures for making this information accessible to people of different cultural, linguistic, and educational backgrounds. For these reasons the Cooper bill scored a 3.5 on this criterion.

The Michel bill required states to develop and implement a health care value information program that would provide price and other information relevant to the purchase of health insurance. However, it allowed states up to six years to develop informational systems that would provide comprehensive comparative information on costs, quality, and outcomes. All information was to be widely distributed in all relevant markets. These too were significant improvements over the current situation, though less fully worked out than Cooper. The six-year delay was unnecessary, and leaving the provisions up to the states meant significant variation around yet unspecified terms. Also, Michel allowed selective marketing and information distribution. Overall, we scored it a 3.0.

The McDermott/Wellstone bill paid little attention to consumer information and education. It did propose placing consumers on various boards, commissions, and the area health councils that would assess the quality and distribution of regional health services. It suggested training outreach workers. It required states and a national quality council to assess the quality of health care being delivered, but it appears that most of it would not have resulted in consumer information. These few initiatives earned the bill a 2.0.

By contrast, the Clinton approach would have provided consumers with extensive information about the quality and outcomes of competing plans. It required that marketing materials be prepared and reviewed for false or misleading information before dissemination. It required both regional and corporate alliances to provide easily understood comparisons of the various health plans, including the results of consumer satisfaction surveys. These "report cards" would have also assessed the outcomes of key services, such as obstetrics or oncology. The bill authorized and funded a comprehensive, age-appropriate school health education program. These provisions earned a 4.5.

Overall, for the second benchmark the four proposals received the following average score:

McDermott/Wellstone	3.3
Clinton	4.0
Cooper	2.0
Michel	0.9

Benchmark 3: Comprehensive and Uniform Benefits

The case for comprehensive and uniform benefits, as well as grounds for exclusion, were made in chapter 3. Equitable access to equitable services assures everyone that their access to opportunities will be restored as much as possible regardless of their health condition or how it may change. A basic or bare bones approach to benefits produces back-door inequities. Likewise, a partial package until money is saved contributes to inequities. Three criteria make up this benchmark: All effective and needed services are to be made affordable and available. Differences in the quality of services and providers, or tiering, are to be minimized. The range of benefits is not to be dependent on "savings" generated elsewhere. Limiting costs is most fair and effective if done from a starting point of universal access to comprehensive services.

Comprehensiveness

A single-payer approach like McDermott and Wellstone's offers a comprehensive package of benefits, including preventive and long-term care services. States and employers can purchase additional benefits. The McDermott/ Wellstone bill gave special attention to the diagnosis and treatment of people with disabilities. It furnished additional services if approved by utilization review. It provided home- and community-based long-term care services for people unable to perform two of five "activities of daily living" tasks without assistance. A national board would have developed practice guidelines and determined which experimental procedures would be included in the national benefit package. Finally, the McDermott/ Wellstone reform recognized the hazards of out-of-pocket disincentives and prohibited them. These features warranted a near-perfect score of 4.5. The Wellstone plan, however, did not treat mental health services with parity to other services.

The heavily managed approach represented by the Clinton bill also mandated a uniform, comprehensive benefit package. All services deemed medically necessary and appropriate by the National Health Board would have been included, with a five-year period for phasing them in. The approach to mental health was to cover inpatient and residential psychiatric treatment only if provided in the least restrictive setting, and only in cases where intensive outpatient treatments were deemed inappropriate. The bill also helped people with severe disabilities pay for community- and home-based services. As well, it proposed a program to help poor children with special needs.

A reform effort like this would normally receive a high score, but various concerns led us to give it a score of 3.5. First, long-term care services were not part of the comprehensive benefit package. Consumers were merely encouraged through tax subsidies to buy private long-term care insurance, which frequently supplies inadequate coverage. Second, not all needed health services were treated the same; mental health and dental would have been phased-in over a longer period of time, if savings permitted. Third, only the severely disabled were eligible for benefits. There were no provisions for people with lesser degrees of disability as there was in the McDermott/Wellstone proposal.

The two market-oriented reforms did not attend to comprehensiveness, though they easily could have. It is difficult, even impossible, to have fair competition without uniform benefits as part of the level playing field, because otherwise the poorer or sicker players become doubly disadvantaged (Enthoven 1988). The more comprehensive the uniform baseline of benefits is, the fairer will be the competition. However, the Cooper bill neither specified the benefits package nor indicated how comprehensive it would be. It postponed these decisions until a Health Care Standards Commission determined which procedures were "medically appropriate." How this would be done was unclear, though procedures in approved clinical trials were singled out for inclusion. Although the Cooper design would have eventually provided nationwide uniformity, little else was clear, and therefore it received a score of 1.5.

The Michel bill also did not specify a set of benefits, except to say that plans must cover essential and medically necessary medical, surgical, hospital, and preventive services. There was no mechanism to assure any uniformity. There seemed no basis for scoring it above the status quo, which is a zero.

These low scores for the market-oriented approaches to reform are particularly disappointing, because there is no reason for competitive markets to take place in the realm of social services under conditions that put some players at a distinct disadvantage to others. There is also an element of negligence, analogous to replacing public school with a private, voluntary market for basic education in which people might or might not attend, and schools might or might not teach basic writing skills. If people do not attend, or attend and do not learn basic skills, the rest of society ends up paying for the consequences in costly, complex, and disruptive ways. Likewise, variable and voluntary coverage of and access to medical services create an unlevel playing field for competition, with costly, disruptive, and complex consequences for society.

Reduced Tiering and Uniform Quality

The second criterion is aimed at reducing the "tiering" by quality differences among competing health plans. The single-payer approach largely avoids the problem because there is only one plan offering only one package of benefits, the same approach that is used in most other countries. It allows individuals full choice of providers, and no one can be discriminated against by the quality of their insurance, because there essentially is no insurance. Yet the McDermott/Wellstone version of the single-payer reform lacked specific measures to assure uniform quality, and we scored it a 3.0.

The heavily managed approach to reform, the Clinton proposal, was weaker on tiers and contained some obstacles to assuring that all patients have access to comparable services. This approach allowed for competition among plans that may charge different premiums. This would probably lead to differences in quality and intensity of care.

To help balance services in its competitive design, the Clinton bill restricted the premiums of the most expensive plans to no more than 120 percent of the average plan. Moreover, plans would receive risk-adjusted payments to help equalize quality across risk groups. Still, low-income individuals and those eligible for subsidies would be less able to afford higher-priced plans, and some stratification would result because higher-priced plans would probably provide better-quality care. Even worse, out-of-pocket expenses would differ, even though premiums would be equalized. Those differences discriminate most severely against the sick and the working class when they can least afford it.

On a more positive note, this proposal would have mainstreamed Medicaid recipients, a significant reduction in present tiering. A number of provisions would have reduced differences in quality, but some serious stratification would remain. We gave it a 2.5.

To be fair, a market approach to reform has to strike a balance between creating a level playing field and rewarding superior performance. The Cooper bill was quite complex from this perspective, or the drafters did not think about their market reform proposal this way. This is our basic point: *the fairness of a proposal must be developed alongside the affordability and the feasibility of a proposal.*

The Cooper bill proposed to abolish Medicaid and replace it with unspecified premium subsidies for enrollment in private health plans. If the premium payments and subsidies for low-income people were inadequate, the health plans would have a financial incentive to provide lower-quality care to them. Low-income individuals would not have been able to afford the other plans because they could only afford the lowest-cost plan, and there was no mechanism for eliminating the stratification among plans. Unlike the Clinton plan, which tried to constrain premium differences, or the McDermott/Wellstone plan, which had none, Cooper proposed no such constraints here. Consequently, inequality would have increased. Lower payments for Medicare might make it more difficult for enrollees to find providers as well. In short, the bill would most likely have resulted in increasingly separate and unequal health plans for the less affluent.

Two redeeming and important features were Cooper's uniform benefits package, once it was phased in, and strong consumer information package. They would help reduce present differences in quality and tiering, and for them we gave the Cooper proposal a 1.5.

The market-based plan of the Michel bill took a laissez faire approach to the market, so there were no provisions for reducing tiers of quality and extra benefits, no uniform benefits package, and not much required market information on price, quality, and performance that would have helped to reduce differences *within* price/benefit tiers, though not *between* them. We think this is an unfair and irresponsible approach to market-based reform. The Michel approach received a zero on this criterion.

Benefits Not Dependent on Savings

The third criterion aims at keeping the benefit package stable even if savings from reform fall below predicted levels. The McDermott/Wellstone and Clinton bills established comprehensive benefits at the outset and made them immune to shortfalls in savings. However, the Clinton bill proposed to improve its mental health benefits in the year 2001 if there were sufficient savings. Consequently, the McDermott/Wellstone bill received a score of 5.0 and the Clinton bill a 4.0 on this criterion.

The Cooper bill did not establish a benefits package until after a five-year phase-in, so its contents would probably reflect savings and costs in the interim. Expanded coverage for prescription drugs and long-term care were explicitly dependent on savings. In a similar fashion, the Michel bill also failed to address this issue adequately. Hence, both bills received a score of zero.

Averaging the scores across all three criteria yields the following results for benchmark 3:

McDermott/Wellstone	4.2
Clinton	3.3
Cooper	1.0
Michel	0.0

Benchmark 4: Equitable Financing—Community-Rated Contributions

No health care reform measure can truly be fair without equitable financing. This requires that the collection of funds be independent of peoples' health status and in proportion to their ability to pay (benchmark 5). This is particularly important because serious health problems or illness fall heavily on only a few people.

As illustrated in figure 4-1, just 2 percent of a population (like a state or county or Blue Cross plan) gets so ill that its treatment consumes 41 percent of all costs (Berk and Monheit 1992). Only 1 percent get hospitalized in a year. And just 10 percent require 72 percent of all costs for their treatment. Moreover, the kinds of people and the kinds of problems that make up that 10 percent keep changing. Thus, any reform that does not attend to the ways in which these people can be discriminated against, and protect them from abuse, is seriously unfair.

A particular favorite of American policy makers is co-payments, which of course discriminate directly against the sick in proportion to how sick they are, up to an annual limit. Contrary to common belief, co-payments do not hold down overall costs but rather transfer costs to the sick from the general pool of people insured (Evans, Barer, and Stoodart 1994; Rasell 1995). Indirectly, exclusion clauses, differences in policy coverage, pay-

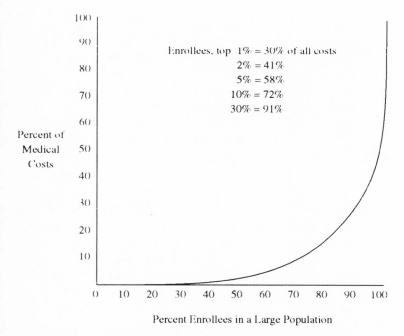

Figure 4–1 Distribution of medical costs across large populations.

ment caps, and waiting periods are forms of de-insurance that also discriminate by health status and do not keep down costs.

This benchmark consists of only two criteria—true community-rated premiums across large populations or taxes and minimal back-door discrimination by risk via out-of-pocket expenditures.

True Community-Rated Premiums

Nearly all universal and fair health care systems collect money through wage taxes or through general taxes. They have nothing to do with people's health status. In the American context, where the "spiral of exclusion" is occurring as private insurers compete for the healthiest people and limit their coverage of the illnesses that their enrollees get, any kind of collection along these lines would get a 5.0. We therefore give the McDermott/Wellstone bill a score of 5.0.

Except for proposals like the McDermott/Wellstone bill, that would collect funds through taxes, most American proposals hedge on "community rating." The term itself has become a verbal football, kicked around to mean several different things. "Demographic community rating," for example, means discrimination by age, sex, and possibly other powerful variables (like social class) that take the premiums far away from equity or the true meaning of community rating. "Community rating by bands" is also not community rating but discriminating by banded classes of people. Another way that community-rated premiums can become less fair is by calculating them for small communities or groups. For example, if each employer used "community rating" for his or her employees, the results would reflect sizeable differences in the age, sex, and occupational risk profile of different companies. To be fair, community rating should be done on a rather large group, of 250,000 or more.

The Clinton bill, representing the heavily managed approach, was a good example of a reform committed to community rating that began to compromise it in the details. The bill called for community rating by plan, but then said it could be adjusted for correlates of health status (such as income, health status, and geographic region) allowed by the National Health Board. The proposal recognized that these two features could stray quite far from true community rating; so it limited how far a plan's premium for providing the required package of services could vary from the premium set by the regional alliance by 20 percent. How unfair provisions like these become would depend heavily on decisions made by the National Health Board.

Even if premiums were based on true community rating, the competing for-profit health plans in this design would probably engage in selective marketing practices and thereby undermine the basic goal of true community-rated contributions. Selective marketing is quite advanced and refined. A familiar indication of how selective health insurance companies could get is provided by the marketing strategies of mail-order catalogues. The same techniques that allow a ski catalogue to be targeted to skiers, and a garden catalogue to be targeted to gardeners, allow insurers to target markets of healthy subscribers. For these reasons, the Clinton plan received a score of 3.5 on the first criterion.

But these observations raise a deeper issue: can equitable contributions be maintained by *any* set of community-rated rules in a market of competing insurers? An important piece of evidence comes from Germany, where hundreds of insurance pools have coexisted for decades with nearly perfect community-rated premiums. They are nonprofit and only implicitly competitive. Yet steadily over time, differentials between the pools grew until today they are the object of a major reform to reequilibrate German health insurance (Wysong and Abel 1990; McGregor 1993).

The lightly managed approach of Cooper to equitable financing was much worse. It allowed health plans to set their own premiums, which could be adjusted for age bands and location, a surrogate for class. It required these risk adjustments to be applied equally to everyone in a plan.

Thus, while the bill prohibited individual underwriting, it allowed limited group risk-adjusted premiums. This looseness promised some improvement over present practices but not much, and therefore the Cooper plan received a score of 2.0.

The market-based proposal of Michel had a similar design, but it also allowed premiums to be adjusted by gender and plan design. This leaves room for many inequities and falls far short of true community rating. It is a slight improvement over current risk rating and therefore received a score of 1.5.

Minimum Discrimination via Cash Payments

The second criterion concerns discriminatory out-of-pocket expenditures. Because the single-payer approach represented by the McDermott/Wellstone bill contained no deductibles or co-payments of any kind, it received a perfect score of 5.0. If there are no out-of-pocket expenditures, this type of back-door discrimination cannot occur.

Under the heavily managed Clinton proposal, all health plans could have varied their deductibles, coinsurance rates, and co-payments. In addition, all plans had to impose co-payments for all out-of-network providers. Alliances would have charged enrollees a 20-percent surcharge for all nonemergency services received outside of its area. Out-of-pocket charges for certain home health services would also have been increased. However, balance billing was not allowed. Regardless of plan, total out-of-pocket expenses were limited to $1500 for an individual and $3000 for a family.

While the disallowance of balance billing and the limiting of out-of-pocket expenditures are commendable, the Clinton plan received a score of only 1.5 because its out-of-pocket provisions were regressive and discriminated against the sick. Since the cheaper plans might have more cost sharing, and since people with disabilities and chronic problems are more likely to have lower incomes, the Clinton design was doubly unfair to these people. Cost sharing would have been greater both absolutely and relatively for them. Marginal and migrant workers, who must travel to find work, would have borne an extra burden from high co-payments for out-of-network providers. So would patients with subtle or complex problems who felt they needed to go outside the network of their managed care provider.

Quite similar features, with similar inequities, were found in the market-based Michel bill and the lightly managed competition Cooper bill. The Cooper bill specified no limit on cost sharing and failed to define the cost-sharing burden for low-income people, leaving these matters up to a commission. This dropped its score from a 1.5 to a 0.5. The Michel bill was worse because it placed no limits on them. It also allowed balance billing and required health plan enrollees to pay more out-of-pocket for using nonparticipating providers for nonemergency care. In short, the Michel provisions made no improvement on the unfair practices today and therefore earned a score of zero.

The low scores of the three plans based on competition seem to reflect the commonly held view that the American health care system suffers from "too much insurance" and that patients must pay more of their bills directly out-of-pocket so that they will become prudent shoppers. From a comparative perspective, this is a strange American belief not supported by the facts. When it comes to medical care, people are not nearly so price sensitive as they are when it comes to buying chicken. Even when they are price sensitive, they cannot do much about it when they have an acute problem and their doctor recommends a specific procedure. The only real shopping they can do is for primary care and elective surgery, which do not account for much of the nation's medical bill nor for the forces that drive medical costs up. We should pay attention to the fact that all of the comparative nations that have held their medical costs in check while providing high-quality, prompt services to everyone have used the opposite approach. They have gotten everyone into a fully insured system and then controlled the costs of that system as a whole. Moreover, as underscored here, out-of-pocket payments are doubly unfair. They discriminate by income and by degree of sickness. In short, a fair competitive system would not be structured around direct payments.

Total average scores for this benchmark are:

McDermott/Wellstone	5.0
Clinton	2.5
Cooper	1.3
Michel	0.8

Benchmark 5: Equitable Financing—By Ability to Pay

Equity in financing also requires that all direct and indirect payments, including out-of-pocket expenses, be scaled to peoples' ability to pay. Premiums and subsidies should be pegged to a broad-based sliding scale of income after taxes, housing, food, and a basic living budget. There should be no abrupt cut-off points.

The single-payer approach to reform represented by McDermott and Wellstone would have collected funds primarily through income and corporate taxes. It also proposed increased taxes for wealthy individuals and corporations, plus a 7.5 percent levy on income tax. Except for those below 120 percent of the poverty rate, people would also have had to pay $65 a month for long-term care insurance. Like most health insurance systems in other countries, this proposal did not allow co-payments, deductibles, or balance billing. These provisions come as close to financing by ability to pay as one could imagine and therefore earned a score of 5.0.

The heavily managed approach represented by Clinton relied on tax-exempt premiums, which are doubly regressive. Flat premiums per person or per family represent a much greater share of an average workers' take-home pay, and the worth of the tax deduction rises with income. Much better is a flat percentage of wages, like current contributions that workers make to Medicare Part B. It is also important to realize that employers' "contributions" largely come out of workers' take-home pay (Reinhardt 1993). What is commonly called a "benefit" is no gift at all.

Another proposal was a cigarette tax. While a substantial tax raises the cost of cigarettes, discourages smoking, and brings in some money for health care, it is important to realize that it is a regressive, inequitable tax. An extra *amount,* like a dollar tax per pack, represents a greater proportion of working class income than middle-class income, while an extra flat *percent* represents the same proportion. Moreover, the less people earn, the more likely they are to smoke. We may decide its benefits outweigh its inequities, but we should openly debate the matter.

Still another proposal was a flat-rate tax for Medicare Part B, which of course would also be regressive, though less so than a cigarette tax. The cost-sharing provisions discussed in benchmark 4 were also highly regressive. The impact of these measures was softened for some classes of lower-income people through some subsidies. Weighing these policy proposals, we decided the Clinton approach was about a 2.0, an improvement over the status quo but well short of equitable financing.

We debated giving this package of policies for raising funds a lower score because of a fundamental problem. Employment itself is becoming de-stabilized. The United States has never had a solid employment structure like Germany, with strong and pervasive unions. It has long had a large underground labor market of people who pick, process, and prepare food, who work in a large variety of sweatshops, and who provide a wide range of services to the middle and upper classes. But in recent years, even the mainstream managerial, technical, and regular markets have been eroded. Constantly, large corporations announce layoffs of thousands of people. Even more get dismissed because of mergers and acquisitions. A growing portion are fired and then rehired through contracting and piecework pay, just so the company can avoid paying any benefits (Ansberry 1993). The temp market has also grown rapidly; there are even temp managers and vice presidents.

These trends cast doubt on the wisdom and practicality of funding health care through employment. They also raise serious questions about how equitable employment-based financing can be. This growing army of just-in-time and underground workers are likely to be either self-insured or uninsured, with complicated patterns of income from different jobs for different periods of a given year. It seems that any proposal founded on employment-based premiums is becoming a way to finance a health care system that is inequitable in terms of all five benchmarks.

The voluntary employment-based approach to funding has even more problems, and they are instructive to review. The Cooper bill is a useful example, because it used a sophisticated, complex approach involving many features that policy makers are still using. Under this bill, employers could pay for some or all of their employees' premiums, but there were no requirements to do so. Ultimately, individuals were responsible for premium payments, but a sliding scale of subsidies were proposed from 200 percent of poverty down. This was helpful, though the subsidies appeared to be smaller than in the Clinton plan. More important, there were no limits on premiums and their differential over time, nor on cost sharing.

The bill did address the tax-favored status of health insurance. It proposed taxing premiums above the lowest cost plan but allowed the self-employed to deduct their premiums fully. It also proposed taxing high-income Medicare recipients on their Part B premiums. The bill required cost sharing, except for preventive services. It provided for some cost sharing for low-income people and some cost-sharing assistance. A Health Care Standards Commission would have developed the specifics for both. These cost-sharing provisions are highly regressive. On balance, we gave this package a score of 1.0.

The market-based plan to reform represented by Michel had proposed an equally open approach to funding, with the same likely inequities resulting. It also expanded Medicaid to cover all those below the poverty line, although it required them to participate in low-tier Health Allowance Programs. The subsidies for people below this income level were not adequately specified, and the state's Health Alliance Program could require participants to pay some or all of the premium and cost sharing based on a sliding scale. States could also subsidize people up to 200 percent of the poverty rate. As part of the applications, states could require means testing, yet there were no guaranteed subsidies for people with income over 100 percent of poverty. The bill set no limits on out-of-pocket expenditures, and the poorest would have to pay some amount for their coverage. Among Medicare recipients, Michel would have taxed the wealthy for their premiums.

Perhaps the most relevant feature for today was Michel's proposal for medical savings accounts (MSAs). These would be tax-free like IRAs to encourage individuals to save so that they would pay for all their medical expenses up to a ceiling, such as $2500 within a year. Employers could provide a catastrophic umbrella policy that would pay for all expenses above the ceiling. They could take their current contribution to health insurance, pay for the catastrophic policy, and give the rest to employees for their MSA. Employers could offer a variety of policies with different ceilings. The higher the ceiling, say $5000, the less the catastrophic policy would cost the employer, so that the balance going to the employee's MSA would be higher. Small employers who now find health insurance unaffordable would be able to buy at least the catastrophic policy as a safety net for any of their employees who becomes seriously ill. This program would be voluntary.

If there were money left over at retirement, it could be rolled over to the person's IRA. The chief results would be that the vast majority of people would be accountable for their own medical expenses, a large amount of current billing costs for small charges would be eliminated, and a lively competitive market would develop among providers to offer patients the best value for their money. The market would be appropriately diverse. People keen on prevention would choose providers who offered comprehensive programs in prevention. People who value house calls would choose providers who offered them, and so forth. Along the way, current tax inequities would be eliminated, and aside from the tax exemption, the program would be privately run.

Many variations of this proposal are possible. For example, the program could be mandatory in some way, though the chosen means would affect its relative fairness. To address the problem of people with illnesses or disorders that consume their MSA every year, one could devise lifetime deductibles for different disorders to replace the annual ceiling.

The medical savings account proposal has many merits over the current way in which private health insurance is paid and structured. Nevertheless, it poses serious forms of unfairness. As proposed by Michel, it would be voluntary, giving it a low score on benchmark 1. Its claim of saving billions in administrative costs is false, because all the small bills would remain, only transferred over to the private cash market of health care services; so it would not improve the current inefficiencies (benchmark 7). Most pertinent to this benchmark, a flat ceiling, like $2500, rather than a ceiling proportionate to income, like 7 percent, would be highly regressive, as illustrated by Figure 3–1 in chapter 3. A fixed amount would put a heavy burden on about 40 percent of the nation's workers. It would cut into their budget for housing, food, and other essentials. By contrast, for the nation's top 20 percent by income, it would hardly affect their lifestyle.

For these reasons, the MSA is most likely to be used by more affluent families, while less affluent families would opt for standard, more comprehensive policies. This would exaggerate an inequity already built into the proposal, that the more affluent one is, the more one can afford a higher deductible and save tax free. The sizeable accumulation over thirty or forty years would then be rolled over into one's IRA as retirement income. The inequitable distribution of serious health problems by income would further exaggerate this inequity. Thus, the working class would use up their MSAs more often. Their medical bills up to the flat ceiling would cast a heavy burden on their household income, and they would be least able to accumulate MSA savings as a second tax-free income after retirement. In short, the MSA proposal as outlined by Michel would contain three forms of inequity by ability to pay that favor affluent employees. We rated the bill a zero on this criterion. Once again, advocates of the market-oriented approach did not think through how to make it equitable.

The scores for this benchmark are:

McDermott/Wellstone	5.0
Clinton	2.0
Cooper	1.0
Michel	0.0

Discussion

This chapter has applied detailed criteria for five benchmarks of fairness for reforming health care insurance to four prominent, highly professional proposals. It illustrates how the criteria can be used to compare the relative fairness of different proposals and to pinpoint which aspects most need improvement. The next chapter will continue with the second five benchmarks, which focus more (but not exclusively) on the reform of health care services.

Overall for the first five benchmarks, the tallies in Table 4-1 are 22.2 out of a possible 25 for Wellstone's bill, 15.8 for Clinton's, 7.1 for Cooper's, and 2.9 for Michel's. One way of regarding these scores is from the status quo, or the level of (un)fairness currently allowed in the American health care system. The two most unregulated reforms in effect regard the status quo as just about right. Given that the current level of fairness in the health care systems in almost any other advanced country would take at least a 4.0 to match, these reform proposals accept a high level of unfairness by the standards of Western civilization at the end of the twentieth century.

These scores could also be regarded in terms of their distance down from a 5.0, that is, from reforms that would enable American health care to manifest the concept of fairness presented in this book. Such reforms would get a perfect score of 100 percent, or an A+. If we multiply the average scores for these proposals by four to convert them into percent-

	Public Financing/ Private Practice (McDermott/Wellstone)	Heavily Regulated Market Approach (Clinton)	Moderately Regulated Market Approach (Cooper)	Least Regulated Free Market Approach (Michel)
Benchmark 1: *Universal Access—Coverage and Participation*				
Mandatory Coverage and Participation	4.5	4.0	1.5	0.5
Prompt Phase-in	4.5	4.0	2.0	1.5
Portability	5.0	4.0	2.0	1.5
Average Score for Benchmark 1	4.7	4.0	1.8	1.2
Benchmark 2: *Universal Access—Minimizing Nonfinancial Barriers*				
Minimizing Maldistributions	5.0	4.5	0.5	0.5
Reform of Health Professional Education	4.0	4.0	4.0	0.0
Minimizing Language, Culture, Class Barriers	2.0	3.0	0.0	0.0
Minimizing Educational and Informational Barriers	2.0	4.5	3.5	3.0
Average Score for Benchmark 2	3.3	4.0	2.0	0.9
Benchmark 3: *Comprehensive and Uniform Benefits*				
Comprehensiveness	4.5	3.5	1.5	0.0
Reduced Tiering and Uniform Quality	3.0	2.5	1.5	0.0
Benefits Not Dependent on Savings	5.0	4.0	0.0	0.0
Average Score for Benchmark 3	4.2	3.3	1.0	0.0
Benchmark 4: *Equitable Financing—Community-rated Contributions*				
True Community-rated Premiums	5.0	3.5	2.0	1.5
Minimum Discrimination via Cash payments	5.0	1.5	0.5	0.0
Average Score for Benchmark 4	5.0	2.5	1.3	0.8
Benchmark 5: *Equitable Financing— By Ability to Pay*	5.0	2.0	1.0	0.0

Explanation of Scores: Reform proposals were judged according to how much they would likely increase or decrease the fairness of the U.S. health care system. A score of zero represents no change from the status quo of 1994. Scores range from −5.0 to +5.0.

ages, the single-payer package received an overall score of 88.4 percent, or a B+ for making health care insurance fair. The heavily managed Clinton bill received a 63.2 percent, or a D for improving fairness. (This may surprise many who think of the Clinton reforms as providing solid universal health insurance; but the proposals scored badly in two related areas: discrimination by income through co-payments and through regressive premiums.) The lightly managed Cooper proposal received a 28.4 percent, or an F; and the market-based Michel bill a 11.6 percent, or an F-, compared to a truly fair system. These scores for the first five benchmarks and the reasoning behind each of the thirteen specific criteria provide much material for discussion.

5

Using the Benchmarks to score Health Care Reforms

Chapter 4 addressed the first five benchmarks and the greater fairness that different reform proposals would bring. This chapter continues with benchmarks 6-through-10 concerning aspects of fairness built into how money is spent, how services are provided, how much choice people have, at what level budgets are set, and the issue that few reform efforts address—how decisions about rationing are done. Once again, we wish to share our thinking as we use the benchmarks to assess real-world reform bills, with all their lapses, overlaps, contradictions, and vagueness. This seems the best way to show how others can put fairness on the table next to affordability and other key criteria for assessing a given reform idea.

These assessments necessarily combine philosophical criteria with sociological and economic research and information about how the health care world treats aspects of a given reform idea. Our scores of benchmarks 6 through 10 depend even more on our understanding of how the health care world works than they did for benchmarks 1 through 5, and therefore our scores are vulnerable to inaccuracies and changes in circumstances. Nevertheless, they take us beyond regarding disputes about the fairness or unfairness of a policy as "differences of opinion" or "political disagreement." They unpack these differences so that people can understand the moral, economic, or social components on which they agree and disagree. This, in turn, facilitates creative and workable solutions.

Roughly speaking, these five benchmarks have to do with how money is allocated and spent, while the first five concerned how money is collected. The two are more separable than many usually think. That is, how a system collects its money is analytically distinct from how it organizes and pays for services. For example, money can be collected through employment contributions, taxes, or individual purchases but then be allocated through government programs, private markets, nonprofit delivery systems, or many other arrangements. We tend to think that if money is collected through taxes, services must be delivered through a government system (single payer); but the tax revenues could buy private managed care services, as in the managed care contracts for Medicare. Conversely, we tend to think that we are used to collecting money through private premiums and then paying individual doctors or health facilities; but the organization of services could be highly structured and regulated, as is happening with managed care delivery systems. The point is for readers to be open-minded about how best to combine fair ways to collect money with fair ways to allocate it and organize services.

Benchmark 6: Value for Money—Clinical Efficacy

This is the first of two benchmarks that concern the great need to reduce clinical and administrative waste before any kind of direct or indirect rationing takes place. Unnecessary procedures or overtreatment, high administrative costs, an emphasis on heroic intervention rather than primary care and prevention, overpricing, and fraud have unfortunately characterized American health care for decades. The wizardry of heroic interventions has prompted fans to call it "the best health care system in the world," but if "the best" system minimizes serious illness from arising in the first place, by providing comprehensive primary care and good public health for everyone, then American health care has a long way to go.

This benchmark's first two criteria gauge a proposal's advancement of primary care, public health, and other forms of prevention. The last two criteria concern systematic outcomes assessments and resource utilization. They gauge the extent to which the proposed reforms assess health care outcomes and quality and minimize both the overutilization and underutilization of resources.

Value for money, especially through clinical efficacy, is critical because doctors and hospitals have tremendous advantages over patients and insurance schemes. The advantages begin with information asymmetry: doctors and hospitals know far more than patients do about the medical problem at hand. Further, doctors advise patients about what to do, and most patients want it that way. Thus the seller (the physician) also tells the buyer (the patient) what she or he needs.

Doctors also have considerable control over what patients and even insurance companies know, because they control what goes into the chart. For some time, consulting firms have been showing physicians and nurses how to write up charts so that the diagnosis is the one that pays the hospital or doctor the most.

Finally, as if those advantages were not enough, much of medicine is contingent and emergent. That is to say, what is done depends on what was tried before and how it worked out, and what is done is not clear until a full clinical picture comes together. Both the emergent and contingent qualities of medicine are in the provider's hands. Choices are often murky, even when there is rigorous research comparing the relative effectiveness of alternate procedures.

Value for money and clinical efficacy are also important because health care markets lack so many of the requirements for effective competition, as shown in table 5–1.

Especially with managed care corporations, there are only a few buyers and sellers, in some areas essentially just one. Very few enter or exit what is rhetorically called a "competitive" market. Rather, a symbiotic relationship develops between the big buyers and the big sellers. Good information on quality, product, and price is scarce or, in some cases, nonexistent. What information that does exist is costly and not easily available to patients. Add to this picture the emergent and contingent character of medicine, together with the control providers have over information and decisions, and it is understandable why most economists over the past fifty years have concluded that medicine simply lacks the basic requirements for a viable and fair market. They call it "market failure," but "failure" does not mean competition breaks down, like a car having engine problems. Rather, it means that providers, managers, or investors can gain power and profits without becoming more efficient or productive, because the market does not work to reward the most efficient or productive. There are much easier ways to "win," as illustrated in table 5–2.

By cornering markets, manipulating data, colluding, using strong-arm tactics against new competitors, or shifting costly patients over to somebody else's budget, institutions can gain in markets that fail to meet the basic requirements for a fair and viable market. Because health care is so skewed, the stakes are high and the potential profits from working the market are immense.

One must realize that imperfect competition is not like imperfect singing that is slightly off-key, or "seconds" in china that have a few tiny imperfections. Rather, if one or more requirements fall away, competition can spin off in any one of several directions away from maximum efficiency and value. Using health services in the most cost-effective ways is thus a critical safeguard against these problems.

Table 5-1   Requirements for Competitive Markets vs. Hazards of Health
Care Markets

Requirements for Competitive Markets	Hazards of Health Care Markets
Transaction and market costs zero.	Large transaction and market costs.
Many buyers and sellers.	Few buyers and/or sellers. Market capture.
Nature, quality, effectiveness, and price of products or service known. No market failure.	Nature, quality, effectiveness, and/or price of products or service somewhat known and variable. Some market failure.
Power, rules, hierarchy don't exist.	Power, rules, hierarchies found everywhere.
Manipulations, gaming, cost shifting unknown.	Manipulations, gaming, cost shifting prevalent. Induced market failure.
Losers collapse, disappear.	Losers stay around. System carries their inefficiencies.
Maximum efficiency.	Maximum inefficiencies.
Responsive to customers.	"Responsive" to customers. Induced demand, product, or service dilution or substitution, misleading information.

Emphasis on Primary Care and on Public Health and Prevention

A strong emphasis on primary care and on public health and prevention are likely ways to decrease the need for and use of costly subspecialty medicine. A proposal that emphasizes these areas is more fair because it keeps people healthy for less money.

American single-payer proposals happen to emphasize primary care. If we use the McDermott/Wellstone bill as representative, it advocated devoting half the medical residencies to primary care within five years and building up an adequate supply of midlevel primary-care providers. The bill proposed an American Health Security Standards Board to develop specific methods for attaining this goal, and it would have reduced payments to any state that failed to achieve it.

The bill also doubled the existing level of grant funding for community-based primary-care facilities and created an Office of Primary-Care and Prevention Research in the National Institutes of Health. The office was to identify and coordinate research on primary care and disease prevention. Perhaps most important, the bill would have reimbursed primary-care providers at a higher rate than specialists (according to staff for the bill). Yet the McDermott/Wellstone approach to single payer did not use primary-care doctors as coordinators. People could go straight to subspecialists if they wanted, and given the American penchant for doing so, they probably would. In short, better pay for primary care would help recruit more doctors into it, but it probably would not affect much how patients behave. The best systems, like HMOs or Britain's National Health Service, provide

Table 5-2   Why Bother Becoming More Efficient or
Productive? (Alternate responses to competition)

How providers are supposed to respond:
• Become more productive by working harder.
• Become more efficient via faster work, reorganized work.

Easier, more profitable, and more likely responses:
• Dominate markets; exclude or crush competitors; set prices.
• Collude among colleagues.
• Have tying relations, which require users of one service to
    use related ones.
• Specialize, which minimizes competition in a market niche.
• Innovate, induce demand, expand markets, corner a niche.
• Elaborate diagnosis or treatment to increase income.
• Upcode or manipulate data to increase revenues.
• Focus on healthier patients or patients with acute, treatable
    disorders.
• Focus on profitable services and drop others.
• Refer costly or troublesome patients to someone else's budget.

excellent primary-care services through a patient's personally chosen physician, who then decides with the patient what specialty services are needed
(Starfield 1993; Fry et al. 1995). This is unfortunately known in the United
States as "gatekeeping," a term that strips away the personal intimacy and
clinical wisdom of a doctor-patient relationship, so that one is left with the
image of the doctor as a sentinel at the gate to specialty care, challenging all
comers.

One of the most promising ways to reconfigure health care is to create
community-based primary-care groups on a capitation basis, which the
McDermott/Wellstone bill proposed. This is important, because it provides
the basis for addressing the patterns of health problems and risk factors in
the twenty-first century within a firm budget. A fee-schedule approach has
the fault of rewarding more procedures and not rewarding innovative con-
figurations of service that provide more value for money. But just how the
capitation for these groups would be carved out of a fee-and-volume budget was unclear. Overall, the McDermott/Wellstone plan earned a 2.0 for
getting more value out of the money spent. A strong approach would
require everyone to choose a primary-care provider, who would then coordinate all their care.

The McDermott/Wellstone approach had some public health measures
and other forms of prevention as well. For example, it increased funding
for Public Health Block Grants by 25 to 50 percent. It called for training
additional community outreach workers. The bill would have also used
public health data to help set service and research goals for disease preven-

tion. The bill failed, however, to fund core public health functions as well as new public health initiatives adequately. The set-aside for public health was only 0.1 percent of total health spending, one-thirtieth of the amount recommended by the American Public Health Association (Feingold 1994). Accidents, secondary prevention (i.e., early detection), and tertiary prevention (i.e., of chronic disabilities and chronic illness) were largely ignored. Also, the public health functions were not grounded in local departments. In sum, the McDermott/Wellstone proposals only somewhat strengthened public health and prevention over the present and thus increased value for money. We decided a score of 1.5 was about right.

How might a heavily managed version of competition score on primary care and prevention? The heavily managed Clinton bill authorized $600 million a year to help educate physicians and nurses in primary care delivery. It provided primary-care physicians with extra compensation from Medicare and a 20-percent payment bonus for practicing in underserved areas. Finally, the bill relied heavily on systems of managed care that significantly reduced the ratio of medical specialists to primary-care providers and acted as filters for specialty care. These measures are superior to McDermott and Wellstone's single-payer version and earned a 4.5. We only have two relatively minor concerns. Primary-care providers were too narrowly defined, and adequate primary care cannot be provided without an adequate public health infrastructure.

Concerning public health, the Clinton bill paradoxically is an example of a bill that has a great deal about public health and yet (based on our analysis) is not strong. It increased funding for core public health activities, such as environmental protection and infectious disease control, to $750 million in its first five years. It made grants available to the states for training public health professionals and educating the public about disease prevention. Money for the latter was to be increased annually by $200 million between 1997 and the year 2000. States could have also applied for additional grants to develop and implement community-based strategies to improve health promotion and disease prevention.

As with McDermott/Wellstone, funding for these and related efforts was inadequate. Accidents, secondary prevention, and tertiary prevention were not adequately addressed. But there was a more basic problem. A competitive approach to holding down costs works against community-based public health and prevention. In an era of chronic disorders and risks, this is a serious weakness; it means that no one competing plan can afford, or is motivated, to be concerned about community-wide risks or health problems. With several plans in an area, and with patients being encouraged to switch plans in response to marketing, no stable, community-based foundation for prevention and public health is possible. These are public goods in a private health care market. Overall, we thought that these public health measures warranted a 2.5 for increasing fairness through greater value.

A lightly managed market approach to health care might or might not emphasize the importance of primary care. For example, the Cooper bill did. It authorized the Health Care Standards Commission to allocate entry-level positions among the nation's medical residency programs based on its needs assessment of primary and specialty care. The bill called for retraining medical specialists to deliver primary care, and it provided additional training to physician assistants, nurse practitioners, midwives, and other allied health professionals. In fact, the bill required that at least 15 percent of the funds available for such training be spent on increasing the number of primary-care providers.

As with the Clinton proposal, these measures addressed both the short-term and long-term need for more primary-care providers. Managed competition greatly increases the use of primary care as the coordinating "gate-keeper" for increasing value for money. No mention, however, was made of paying primary-care providers more. This is an important issue because they are now compensated much less than surgeons and subspecialists. Overall, we concluded that the Cooper approach is slightly less effective than Clinton and earned a 4.0.

Concerning public health and prevention, the Cooper approach to reform based on markets extended the present public health system and other forms of prevention. It expanded several public health programs, such as those for tuberculosis, AIDS, cancer and cigarette smoking, and the Office of Disease Prevention and Health Promotion. The bill authorized some new money for these expansions, but again the sums were relatively small. It broadened preventive services under Medicare to include colorectal screening, some immunizations, mammography, and well-child care. Preventive services would be the only ones exempt from deductibles or co-payments.

The Cooper bill approach to lightly managed competition showed an awareness of how much all competitors and society as a whole can gain by preventing as much disease and dysfunction as possible before services are needed. Several public health programs, however, were extended without adequate funding, only $700 million for a three-year period. Core public health functions, such as environmental protection, were not funded at all. Two increasingly important public health issues—chronic illness and violence—were likewise omitted. Again, accidents, secondary prevention (i.e. early detection), and tertiary prevention (i.e. of chronic disabilities and chronic illness) were not sufficiently discussed. Moreover, some of the bill's "proposals" reauthorized what already existed. For example, it reauthorized existing public health programs and grants, which were not going to expire anytime soon. On balance, we gave it a 2.0 for strengthening public health in several ways but at low levels of funding.

The market-based approach to reform represented by groups like the Heritage Foundation and the Michel bill appear to foster primary care through the benefits of competition. But since their version of competition is unmanaged and people can choose to go to subspecialists as they do now, value for money through primary care may or may not be increased. It would depend on how the unmanaged market configured over time. Beyond this general observation, the Michel bill made small gestures towards good ideas that seemed almost puzzling. For example, it called for federal grants to bolster outpatient primary care in underserved areas but then restricted them to no more than $100,000 for no longer than a year, hardly enough to make a difference. Moreover, these funds could only be used to *coordinate* the delivery of services, not deliver them. This seemed hardly worth the bother. Likewise, the bill encouraged physicians to volunteer practicing in medically underserved areas but with nothing to back it up.

Slightly more substantial, the bill increased the funding for community and migrant health centers by $1.5 billion over a five-year period, a relatively small amount spread over a relatively long period of time. To increase the supply of primary-care providers, the bill called for the retraining of physicians and the additional training of physician assistants but with no authorized funding. These weak measures plus some market effect earned the Michel proposal a 1.0. Otherwise, the Michel bill featured special programs for rural hospitals and emergency services, both of which enhance specialty services delivered after a medical problem has become serious, rather than early management of risk and treatment through primary care.

Concerning public health and prevention, the Michel version of unregulated market reform extended the present public health infrastructure with some new money, but not nearly the amount recommended by the American Public Health Association. Core public health functions, such as environmental protection, were not funded. In fact, departments of public health were not even mentioned. There was also no funding for violence protection. Accidents, secondary prevention, and tertiary prevention were neglected. Medical injuries was the only area of prevention dealt with by the bill. It required that all health care providers participate, at least once every three years, in a program specifically designed to reduce patient injuries, supported by grants and technical assistance from the Secretary of Health and Human Services. These equally thin efforts earned the Michel bill a 1.0.

Systematic Assessment of Outcomes and Minimizing
Overutilization and Underutilization

The need for systematic assessment of services strikes us as ubiquitous, something that all approaches to reform need. One obvious way to address it is to establish and fund an institution dedicated to it. The McDermott/ Wellstone version of the single-payer approach, for example, would have created a ten-member American Health Security Quality Council to collect outcomes-research data and use it to develop practice guidelines. The council would use these guidelines to identify practitioners delivering poor-quality care and develop procedures to help rectify the problem. The bill required each state to assess the quality of its health care delivery systems according to federal guidelines. States could establish utilization review programs and deny payment to services not approved by these programs.

To help facilitate quality assessments, all patient records would become part of a uniform electronic data base. Moreover, the McDermott/Wellstone bill more than doubled existing levels of funding for this type of research. These reforms earned a score of 4.5, flawed only because there was less than perfect integration among the various assessments, across regions, and between clinical and financial data.

Concerning improved resource allocation, the McDermott/Wellstone bill contained some measures specifically designed to control utilization and improve resource allocation. For example, it encouraged the creation of multidisciplinary practices, called Community Health Service Organizations, and employed Medicare volume-performance standards. Both would have improved overall quality of care. To address the problem of overutilization, the bill employed managed care and global budgets to discourage unnecessary services. To combat the danger of underutilization, the bill called on health care providers to develop standards of appropriate care based primarily on patient needs, and not on financial concerns. The Quality Council would develop "standards for education and sanctions" to punish consistent providers of poor-quality care. These reforms earned a score of 4.0. They represent major advances over the situation in 1993, though safeguards against the real dangers of underutilization did not seem sufficiently strong. The reforms also left too much variation from state to state.

The heavily managed competition approach to reform represented by the Clinton proposal made similar recommendations, though with different details. They would have received a score of 4.5 as well, except for one major difference. The McDermott/Wellstone approach to reform controlled price to the customer through negotiated fee schedules and budgets so that choice was focused mainly on quality. This is the way that most national health care systems do it. But all three versions of reform through managed competition under review here focused on competition by price as well. Under such an arrangement, quality is likely to cost more. As a result, quality will vary by income, which is considerably more unfair than if it does not. Having plans compete to see which can provide the best care at the same price is also more likely to increase value for money than having plans compete for quality where they can raise prices. Value for money may also be less because patients judge quality largely by the price of service. Nevertheless, the Clinton approach offered several improvements over the status quo and therefore earned a 3.5.

Concerning utilization control and resource allocation, the heavily managed approach to competition represented by the Clinton bill required that clinically relevant guidelines be established, reviewed, and updated to help health care providers treat their patients more effectively and appropriately. It proposed establishing a national clearinghouse to disseminate these practice guidelines broadly. In addition, the bill called for regional professional foundations to help providers improve their delivery of health services. The sharp reduction in fee-for-service medicine would probably have reduced the overutilization of resources. To deal with consumer complaints concerning quality of care, the bill required each alliance to have an ombudsman and each health plan to have grievance procedures. Most important, physician profiling and market competition with widely disseminated information on comparative price and quality would be used to minimize both over- and underutilization.

These recommendations would significantly reduce inequities in current services and earned a 4.0. In this era of managed care, the principal threat to the quality of care is underutilization, which is difficult to detect and most likely to harm the least well-off. A excellent comparative data reporting system would help a great deal because of "the Edsel effect": Any provider group that becomes known for inferior quality will lose customers rapidly and then have to spend years earning back a good reputation.

The lightly managed approach to competition represented by the Cooper bill aimed to reduce inequities that stemmed directly or indirectly from problems of clinical efficacy. It also began with an Agency for Clinical Evaluations to assess systematically diagnostic procedures and clinical treatments. The agency was to share its findings with health care providers and establish a national health data system to facilitate its assessments. This proposal, however, contained much less detail than the first two. There was no authorized funding and no time frame. While these are serious shortcomings, the Cooper plan was clearly focused on improving clinical outcomes and therefore earned a 2.5.

Concerning the criterion of resource utilization, the Cooper bill proposed a national Benefits, Evaluations, and Data Standards Board. It would evaluate the services provided by health plans and set minimum standards of care with the Health Care Standards Commission. The bill required that all approved health care plans meet these standards. To handle enrollees' complaints, the bill obliged each purchasing cooperative to have an ombudsman. Like Clinton, Cooper had a strong system for assessing, comparing, and publishing the performance of different plans and providers that should monitor both over- and underutilization. It also prohibited health plans from operating physician incentive programs that used financial incentives to reduce care to enrollees. These are excellent ideas that anyone can use.

The Cooper plan did have a few weaknesses. It did not adequately address the covert forms of underutilization brought on by managed care systems. It advocated cost sharing, which we have already described in chapter 4 as having several drawbacks and few advantages. Cooper's emphasis on cost sharing, however, was no worse than present practices, and his other proposals would have substantially improved the ability of employers, government programs, and patients to choose plans that provided the best value for money. We gave this package a 3.5.

As a free market approach without governmental interference, the Michel bill was also strong on comparative analysis of clinical efficacy. As an example of good market design making the system more fair, it required all health plans participating in the state Health Allowance Program to have internal quality assurance programs that met standards sponsored and enforced by the state. These standards included uniform reporting of patient satisfaction and clinical data, ongoing monitoring, corrective measures, and annual evaluations. In addition to the latter, these quality assurance programs were to be evaluated annually by an independent, nongovernmental review organization.

Unfortunately, the Michel bill required this system only for providers participating in the low-income plan that concerned the government, as though the government needs help getting good comparative market information on product, quality and price but the largest private market does not. The past fifteen years attest to how poorly the world's large private market in health care faired in getting good market information out to customers. Systematic information comparing price and quality is only now available in some markets. Why not set up this system for all buyers and sellers, not just for government-related ones? In addition, Michel's market information programs would have taken place at the state level, so that significant variations (and confusion) could arise across states. In a highly mobile country, a state approach is a second serious weakness, and therefore the Michel approach earned a 2.0.

To minimize both the overutilization and underutilization of health care resources, the Michel's bill offered the same proposals it did for quality assessment—comparative information about providers and plans within the state low-income plan. We gave it a 2.0 for these proposals as well.

The total average scores for this benchmark are:

McDermott/Wellstone	3.0
Clinton	3.6
Cooper	3.0
Michel	1.5

Benchmark 7: Value for Money—Financial Efficiency

Fair reforms would seek to minimize the costs of health care so as to maximize the amount actually produced and delivered. More specifically, benchmark 7 has four criteria: minimize administrative overhead, employ tough contractual bargaining with all providers and suppliers, minimize cost shifting, and have strong anti–abuse and fraud measures.

Minimizing Administrative Overhead

The single-payer approach represented by the McDermott/Wellstone bill that relies on negotiated fee schedules and budgets would minimize administrative overhead that now consumes about 23 percent of all health care dollars. The bill would have eliminated the main sources that make administrative costs in the American system much higher than in other countries: thousands of different policies and forms; thousands of different insurance companies with different procedures; elaborate, elusive and ever-changing techniques for disputing claims, delaying payments or denying them; and all the administrative armatarium that hospitals and providers have had to assemble to cope with or fight this situation. Uniform, electronic records and billing would be done by large fiscal agents chosen by competitive bidding. These reforms earned a score of 5.0.

The heavily managed approach represented by Clinton would have greatly reduced the range of policies, set national standards, and established a uniform data system. It would also have reduced the number of insurance companies by about 90 percent and routinized billing. At the same time, the number of administrative staff now needed by hospitals, doctors' offices, laboratories, and clinics would have been greatly reduced.

Managed competition is administratively complex, though less complex than the kinds of fragmented, unmanaged markets that have long characterized American health care. In order to deal with the complexities of managing competition, the Clinton reforms proposed health alliances as a new, large layer of bureaucracy. The reforms would have moved Medicaid patients from administratively less costly programs to managed care plans, though these plans might have saved money by managing services better than Medicaid does now. Overall, gains in managerial efficiency in the Clinton design were considerable but still more complex than most other countries, and they earned a 3.0.

Cooper's approach to lightly managed competition also reduced many of the current administrative inefficiencies through standardization of benefits and a comprehensive data system. It proposed that health care be provided by what he called "accountable health plans" (AHP), which would be large managed care networks and some fee-for-service delivery systems. It prohibited health plans from offering supplemental coverage that competed directly with the uniform set of effective benefits. The Cooper bill used tax incentives and the relaxation of federal antitrust laws to encourage providers and insurance companies to form AHPs. It called on the Health Care Standards Commission to coordinate among HPPCs, monitor antitrust issues, and collect electronically all data and claims in standardized form.

The Cooper design also established one Health Plan Purchasing Cooperatives (HPPC) per area to help small businesses and individuals on a voluntary basis buy health insurance. A HPPC was to use only the equivalent of 1 percent of premiums for operating expenses. The bill eliminated Medicaid, which had other benefits, but would lead to greater administrative costs. Also, many more insurance companies would continue under Cooper than Clinton. These proposals were slightly less effective, we thought, than Clinton's, and we gave it a 2.5. We should note the important argument by advocates of managed competition that its somewhat costly management more than pays for itself by reducing utilization. This suggests there is some tension between the empirical assumptions underlying benchmarks 6 and 7, as we noted in chapter 3.

The market-based approach represented by the Michel bill left far more of the current administrative inefficiencies intact. It did, however, require uniform data entry and electronic data transmission, claims processing, and patient billing. It called for using magnetized ID cards and establishing a national clearinghouse for primary and secondary payer information. It proposed combining Medicare Part A and Part B within five years. These are all gains over the current situation, and yet they would have left a system with many policies, many benefits packages, and thousands of insurers to use their techniques for delaying claims that run up such a high administrative bill. Therefore, the Michel reforms earned a 2.0.

Tough Contractual Bargaining and Minimizing Cost Shifting

Any reform proposal can pay attention to these big obstacles in the American system to cost-effective health care, but the four bills we are reviewing here for illustrative purposes varied in how much they built in measures for tough bargaining and no cost shifting. The McDermott/

Wellstone single-payer approach required each state to employ cost-containment measures such as state-level review of capital projects and negotiated fee schedules and global budgets for hospitals and nursing homes. These have been among the most effective tools used by countries like Japan, Germany, and Holland, which have held expenditures to a consistent percent of their GNP over the past fifteen years. The bill proposed a limited rate of return for all profit-making facilities within a state. It also used global budgets for some home and hospice care, long-term care, community-based primary-care, and facility-based outpatient care services. Fee schedules, capitation, and other forms of prospective payments were to be used to pay the rest. The fee schedule for individual practitioners would be based on RBRVS, the relative value scale developed at Harvard for Medicare. To ensure that payments to all practitioners conformed to the budget, it used a German idea, to adjust fees quarterly for changes in service volume. Prices for prescription drugs, approved devices and equipment, and all other items would be negotiated for large volume discounts. On tough bargaining, McDermott and Wellstone's approach earned a 5.0.

By having only one buyer of health care in a region or state, the single-payer model eliminates cost shifting among payers. There would simply be no other payer to shift to, though the McDermott/Wellstone approach would have had corporate alliances as well, and providers could still transfer costs or play "hot potato" with expensive cases among themselves. But the absence of any co-payments and deductibles would eliminate cost shifting to consumers. In addition, the national budget would have distributed money to the states based on their actual costs and the health status of their residents. Community-based primary-care facilities could have received enhanced reimbursements to cover ineligible patients. This design warrants a score of 5.0 for eliminating cost shifting.

Managed competition is designed to strengthen the bargaining power of employers and other payers. The heavily managed approach of the Clinton bill called for extensive market information, active role of the alliance in structuring markets, and competing plans in each area in order to facilitate tough bargaining with minimal cost shifting. The bill required that within a year Medicare Part B use competitive bidding for services and supplies, with the Secretary of Health and Human Services empowered to firmly negotiate if true price competition did not work. This seems likely because competition would center around a handful of large managed care plans, and the anticipated competition would be blunted by the oligopolistic interests of the major players. Moreover, the buyer—whether a regional or corporate health alliance—would be too dependent on any one plan to be tough. As a result, there would be little or no exit out of or entry into the market. Allowing providers to sign up with more than one plan would also dilute the competitive model because providers would essentially be competing against themselves.

Perhaps anticipating the resourcefulness of providers and other sellers to resist cost-containment efforts, evident over the past twenty years, the Clinton proposal had back-up controls such as premium caps. The bill also contained specific cost-control measures for health care providers, drug manufacturers, and Medicare. For example, each plan had to control payments to providers in some way, such as fee schedules. These schedules would apply equally to all providers, whether they participated in the plan or not. If a plan exceeded its budget, payments to all providers would be reduced.

This design of an oligopoly with administered prices supporting it would increase value for money but has the flaws mentioned and is complex with many possible loopholes. We scored it a 3.5 for significant improvement.

To help minimize cost shifting, the Clinton bill required all health plans in an alliance to compete for enrollees. The health plans would receive risk-adjusted payments, and balance billing would not be allowed. Plans would have uniform benefits and payment caps. Mandated universal coverage would result in relatively little uncompensated care. Health care providers would be paid the same regardless of whether they were in or out of a health plan. These provisions earned a 3.0, a significant improvement but open to the inequities of cost shifting that occur through co-payments, deductions, and somewhat regressive premiums.

The lightly managed approach of the Cooper bill contained no provisions for tough bargaining except relatively unmanaged competition. This is the kind of competition the nation has tried for the past fifteen years, and it has reduced the rise of health care expenditures in only a few places for a limited time. (Aaron and Schwartz 1993; Rice, Brown, and Wyn 1993; Enthoven 1993). The bill prohibited states from interfering with the financial negotiations between health plans and their providers. Its commission was prohibited from creating or enforcing any kind of cost controls. Thus, tough cost controls were explicitly forbidden. There were no specified provider payment mechanisms; and no limits were placed on payments. The small-business reforms around HPPCs were voluntary and probably no more effective than the concerted efforts made under a program sponsored by the Robert Wood Johnson Foundation. Thus, the proposed reforms received a score of zero, because they would not have improved the status quo.

On the other hand, the Cooper bill did contain some relatively effective anti-cost-shifting measures. For example, it required "community-rated" premiums for similar plans, though these premiums could be adjusted for location and age. It prohibited experience rating, balance billing, and cost sharing above the amounts specified by the Health Care Standards Commission. It required that a uniform package of benefits be set at the national level. The bill also restricted Medicare spending.

These measures have some serious flaws, however. First, since there were no business or individual mandates to purchase health insurance, there was no guarantee that the amount of uncompensated care would be reduced. If it was not, there would have been little or no reduction in cost shifting. Second, except for preventive services, cost-sharing was required, which disproportionately moves costs to poorer and sicker people. Third, businesses were not required to pay any part of their employees' health insurance. Since they had a strengthened financial incentive not to, they would most likely have continued to shift these cost onto workers. Harris Wofford (1994) cited the *New York Times* as stating that a family earning $30,000 a year would have to spend $5,000 a year for basic coverage. Fourth, the reduction in Medicare spending would put those costs onto other payers. Fifth, since there would have been no universal coverage and no uniform rates across health plans, cost shifting would no doubt have continued, if not escalated. Finally, balance billing was prohibited for those people who would be covered by the act. The strengths and weaknesses of these anti-cost-shifting measures received a score of only 2.0.

The market approach of conservatives as represented by the Michel bill offered three pertinent but marginal proposals to promote tough contractual bargaining. It did not allow states to interfere with the financial negotiations between health plans and their providers. It made individuals more cost conscious by allowing them to establish tax-free medical savings accounts for medical expenses. Third, states could not depend on receiving any more federal dollars for their Health Alliance Program to assist the poor than they would have without the program.

Overall, the market-based Michel approach to reform did not address the need for tough bargaining, and when it did, it discriminated against the least advantaged. As discussed before, unmanaged competition allows many ways for sellers and middle men to profit from forms of market failure. There were no limits on prices or profits, even though market failure characterizes many health care markets (Light 1993). These reforms would not improve the present situation and received a zero.

The Michel bill contained no reforms designed to minimize cost shifting. The issue was simply not addressed. Consequently, it received a score of zero on this criterion too.

Anti–Fraud and Abuse Measures

These two measures for increasing value for money also are independent of any given approach or ideology. One would think that any kind of well-designed health care system would want to minimize fraud and abuse. Yet the four proposals reviewed here differed in the degree to which they addressed them.

The single-payer approach of the McDermott/Wellstone bill required each state to have an independent prevention control unit and an antifraud database to check providers' qualifications and ownership of health care facilities or services. Providers found guilty could be fined, jailed, and/or excluded from the national health care system. These measures are useful, but the bill did not require states to carry them out. They contained no whistle-blower protection or malpractice reform, and they could be unduly influenced by the providers of mainstream medicine. Because of these omissions, the McDermott/Wellstone bill received a score of 3.0 for substantial but not complete improvement over the status quo.

Under the heavily managed approach to competition represented by the Clinton bill, fraud and abuse received serious attention. The bill required the Secretary of Health and Human Services and the Attorney General to establish a national program to coordinate and facilitate enforcement efforts, for which the bill authorized funds. It required each health plan to have an ombudsman office to handle complaints and safeguard patients against abuses. It punished people convicted of fraud, abuse, and other health care crimes by excluding them from participating in health plans and Medicare for five years. They could be liable for civil penalties as well. The bill also restricted self-referrals and kickback schemes. It criminalized various forms of health care fraud, including inappropriate uses of the health security card. These strong measures earned a 3.5, because they overlooked a major area of covert reductions in service and contractual abuse of clinicians by insurance companies. The bill was also not strong on malpractice reform and whistle-blower protection.

The lightly managed approach represented here by the Cooper bill contained relatively few measures specifically designed to reduce abusive and fraudulent behavior on the part of providers and payers, especially the insurance companies. It also had weak enforcement mechanisms, no definition of terms, and no protection for whistle-blowers. Its uniform health claim forms and identification numbers, however, would help significantly. It also required each health plan to have an adequately prepared ombudsman to respond to enrollees' complaints about abuses. We gave these measures a score of 2.0.

The Michel bill's anti–fraud and abuse measures were considerably stronger and showed that a free enterprise approach to reform can be tough on unfair practices when it wants. The bill authorized additional funds to detect and investigate health care fraud. It established an Anti–Fraud and Abuse Trust Fund to help pay for these activities. All fines and other monetary penalties would be deposited in it. It authorized the Attorney

General to pay a person up to $10,000 for information about possible fraud or abuse. It made guilty parties liable for treble damages, forfeiture of property, and restitution payments to injured third parties. In short, the bill significantly strengthened the penalties for health-related fraud or abuse. The bill included private mail carriers in the federal mail fraud statute, better coordinated federal, state and local law enforcement efforts, and it provided greater protection for whistle-blowers.

Like other proposals, the Michel bill would have required most health care providers and payers to have uniform data entry and electronic data transmission, claims processing, and patient billing. The requirement that Social Security numbers be used to process all medical claims would increase administrative efficiency, but it would also reduce fraud and abuse. These proposed reforms receive a score of 3.5. Although they lacked an ombudsman and did not give enough attention to abuses of payers and insurers, they were excellent.

To sum up, the total average scores for this benchmark are:

McDermott/Wellstone	4.5
Clinton	3.3
Cooper	1.7
Michel	1.4

Benchmark 8: Public Accountability

Health care affects fundamental aspects of individual well-being, and institutions that make such important decisions should make them in publicly accountable ways. People must know how the health plans and providers are performing. They must know how resource allocation decisions that affect them are made, and they must have effective procedures for appealing such decisions. While all these decisions and procedures must be publicly accountable, they must also respect patient confidentiality. Accordingly, we scored this benchmark on the basis of four criteria: (1) availability of explicit, public, and detailed procedures for evaluating plans and practitioners; (2) explicit and democratic procedures for allocation decisions; (3) fair grievance procedures; and (4) protection of privacy.

Even though rationing is on the minds of all reformers, none of them gives this critical benchmark for accountability and rationing nearly the attention it deserves. The general strategy is to use doublespeak. A given plan will ration some programs, like Medicare and Medicaid, while at the same time claiming that the reform avoids either rationing or new taxes. We had to hunt to find even a few possibly relevant features of the plans.

Moreover, a zero, or the status quo, is in this case very low compared to other national systems. Except for some legislative acts, there is virtually no public accountability for how health care gets rationed in the United States.

Explicit Public Procedures for Evaluation

Bills were strongest on this criterion of the benchmark because of their data requirements. The McDermott/Wellstone bill would have put consumers on District Health Advisory Councils and would have charged them with assessing the quality and distribution of health care services in a geographical area. Outcomes research would have been gathered nationally and used to develop practice guidelines. States would have been required to review delivery systems in light of these guidelines. The McDermott/ Wellstone bill required states to establish utilization review programs, which would deny coverage and payment for services they did not approve.

These are good ideas that any state or national health care reform effort can adopt. We gave them a score of 4.0. These measures assure public accountability in the process of evaluating health care delivery, but there was little explicitly said about public reporting of evaluations beyond the district councils.

The heavily managed approach to competition represented by the Clinton proposal would have established a detailed and extensive system for gathering, analyzing, and publishing information about the performance of plans and providers. The Secretary of Health and Human Services would have conducted a separate evaluation of ongoing long-term care demonstration projects. These too are excellent ideas, and we gave the package a score of 4.5. They could have been more detailed, but they are a major advance over the present in allowing matters of distributive justice to be based on solid, accessible information.

The lightly managed approach to competition represented by the Cooper bill also established a detailed and extensive system for gathering, analyzing, and publishing information about the performance of plans and providers that we have described before. It received a 3.0 because it was unclear what kind of evaluations would be done of health plans provided by employers who did not obtain insurance through the purchasing cooperatives. It also prohibited states from interfering with utilization reviews by plans so that despite an extensive evaluation system, it was not clear what different plans would have done. Comparative assessment would be weakened.

The market approach of the Michel bill also established a system of evaluation like those already described. It earned a 2.5 because of the long, six-year time frame for states to develop systems of evaluation. The bill also deferred details about reporting to the development of those systems.

Oddly enough, it allowed states to set up the systems but then prohibited them from interfering with the utilization reviews, which would be done only by the health plans. Finally, the bill required the federal government's evaluation program to report its findings to Congress but not to the public.

Explicit Democratic Procedures for Resource Allocation

The second criterion requires fair and democratic decision making at all levels in the health care system concerning resource allocation, especially on limiting the use of beneficial medical services. With respect to the latter, fairness requires that the parties most affected by these rationing decisions be reasonably represented and that the process carefully gather information about costs and effectiveness, weigh the relative value of competing resource allocations, and assess the distributive implications of decisions made. In addition, the process should be at all times publicly accountable. Unfortunately, proponents of all plans were unwilling to admit the need for publicly accountable rationing mechanisms. Apparently, each feared the charge that their proposal would bring rationing, which the others claimed to avoid—a reinforcing circle of denial.

The McDermott/Wellstone bill proposed an American Health Security Standards Board to govern the national program. Its seven members would be appointed by the president. There would also be a twenty-one member consumer advisory council appointed by the board to assist it. There would be similar advisory councils to assist the states. We scored this at 2.0. Although consumers would have been directly involved in decision making, the process itself was not adequately defined. In other words, it was not clear exactly how democratic and publicly accountable the process would be. There was also no recognition of the need to make decisions about limiting the use of beneficial services in an explicit and publicly accountable fashion. Perhaps these bodies would have provided some guidance about limits and resource allocation; but since such guidance was not mandated, it might not happen.

The Clinton bill also established a seven-member national board, appointed by the president, to oversee the implementation and running of the national system. For example, it would have had primary responsibility for setting premium caps and modifying the benefits package in light of changing technology. At the state level, a board of directors with equal numbers of employers and employees would have governed the regional alliances. The Clinton bill called for the governor of each state to appoint an advisory group to assist the state in developing its health plans. Anyone in the state could be eligible, and public hearings would have to be part of the decision-making process. Corporate alliances were to be accountable directly to the Secretary of Labor.

The Clinton bill also received a score of 2.0. There was no requirement that health plans, health alliances, or the national board establish publicly accountable procedures for the rationing of care. The relevant boards were not democratically structured, and their decisions were not easily reviewed or debated by the public. Consumer representatives need sufficient resources to be equal partners in the decision-making processes of these boards. Regional alliances were more accountable than corporate alliances, which had no boards with consumer members. Like McDermott/Wellstone, the bill lacked specificity, and it was impossible to know what kind of democratic process and public accountability would have characterized the decision-making process. As always, vagueness hurts a score.

The Cooper bill proposed a Health Care Standards Commission to oversee its enactment, with its five members appointed by the president. Each HPPC would report directly to the commission but would be run by a cooperative board appointed by the governor. The commission would establish a national package of benefits. States would determine the health plans' service areas. The health plans would be responsible for the delivery of services.

This design shows almost no awareness of the need for fair procedures for allocation and rationing. Perhaps it assumes such decisions will all be done by "the market." If the market were perfect, then all such decisions would be fully informed, open, and democratic (in an economic sense); but health care is far from this ideal. The Cooper approach therefore received a score of 0.5. First, the commission would have enormous power, yet would have only five members who were appointed, remote, and probably not typical consumers. Second, the decision-making processes of the Health Standards Commission and the health plans were completely unspecified and would probably develop in undemocratic, indirect, and unaccountable ways. Would the meetings be open to the public? Would documents be made available? Would the public have the right to speak? In short, these proposals failed to address the issues.

The Michel bill contained no relevant procedures and therefore received a zero. For example, there was no specified consumer or public role in matters of governance. Consequently, all decision-making power would get concentrated in the hands of providers and payers, as it is now. There would be no uniform benefits package, the contents of which would not be a matter for public discussion.

Fair Grievance Procedures

The third criterion concerns fair grievance procedures for both practitioners and patients. Again, this is something that any proposal of any political stripe can and should address. In particular, patients should be able to complain about treatments denied them as a result of resource allocation decisions and have legitimate complaints promptly rectified. Procedures should be consumer friendly. While many lawsuits no doubt lack merit, most do not. Fair grievance procedures would reduce the former while encouraging the latter.

The single-payer proposal by McDermott/Wellstone had no explicit provisions for consumer-type complaints, despite consumer participation in the governing bodies. No ombudsman was required, and there is no provision for malpractice reform. With respect to providers, states would have to establish an appeals process for financial grievances. For this last provision and the influence of consumers on governing boards we thought the bill deserved a score of 1.0.

The heavily managed competition bill by Clinton took on the issue of grievance full force. It required each alliance to have an ombudsman to address problems in the alliance and the health plans. Each plan was also to have grievance procedures for both consumers and providers. Standards for such procedures would be set by the National Health Board. Alliances would also have dispute resolution procedures to resolve financial disagreements. Each state was required to establish and maintain a complaint review office. The bill also included modest malpractice reform. For example, the bill required a nonbinding alternative dispute resolution system, certificates of merit, and limits on contingency fees. Compared to the status quo, we thought these proposals earned a 5.0.

The Cooper version of lightly managed competition also required purchasing cooperatives to have ombudsmen with sufficient salary and staff. It required each health plan to have effective procedures for hearing and resolving enrollees' grievances. It required states to develop alternative dispute resolution procedures and to require that any malpractice suit first go through it. The bill also reduced awards for noneconomic damages, tightened statutes of limitation, and restricted contingency fees. These measures earned a score of 4.0, a substantial improvement, but there were no grievance procedures for providers, and the bill's malpractice reforms were not consumer-friendly. For example, there were several limits on contingency fees, and if the plaintiff loses, he or she pays the expenses of the defense.

The market-based Michel bill largely ignored the issue of grievance. It had no grievance procedures to address most resource allocation concerns, though it did mandate ombudsmen. Only plans contracting with the state were required to have grievance procedures. The bill required medical liability claims to be resolved initially through an alternative dispute resolution system, which every state would have. Other mandated malpractice reforms included limits on defendant's liability, limits on noneconomic damages and attorney's fees, and, in some cases, higher standards of proof. To discourage frivolous lawsuits, the bill required plaintiffs who lost their suit to pay the defendant's legal fees. We scored the Michel bill 2.0 for its limited measures. The alternative dispute resolution provisions earned this bill some credit, but the absence of grievance procedures other than malpractice precluded a higher score.

Adequate Privacy Protection

The fourth and final criterion of this benchmark concerns adequate privacy protection. This too is a way to make a health care system more fair regardless of political orientation. Privacy protection is heightened as an issue, because all four bills required much more extensive and standardized data gathering systems than at present. While these advance benchmarks 6 through 8, they also pose a threat to privacy. Everyone in the country would be carrying an unsecured health security card, with few or no safeguards in place. There could be much opportunity for abuse. The single-payer approach as represented by the McDermott/Wellstone bill recognized this problem but offered no specific solutions. Instead, it called for a national board to develop privacy protection standards. This is a good example of a proposal that vaguely promises to address a problem, somehow, sometime in the future. Overall, the McDermott/Wellstone bill would have made privacy protection more difficult than at present and therefore earned a −1.0. The quandary posed by needing standardized comparative data while opening a Pandora's box of privacy issues needs to be addressed more fully and specifically.

The Clinton bill also recognized the problem, and like McDermott and Wellstone, it mandated a national board to submit detailed proposals for privacy protection legislation. This too is a vague promise of a solution sometime in the future. However, the bill explicitly called for establishing a National Privacy and Health Data Advisory Council, and it had more thoughtful details. Enrollees in the health plans would have the right to know what information was known about them and correct any errors. Health plans would also be required to have an ombudsman and other safeguards to protect enrollees' rights and reduce abuse. The greater specificity and efforts to provide safeguards, weighed against a basically greater threat to privacy than at present, led to a score of 1.0.

The Cooper bill addressed the issue of protecting privacy with greater urgency but less detail. It insisted that within six months, a national commission must develop and implement privacy protections. However, the bill contained no details and no sanctions. Weighing the basically greater threat to privacy against an unspecified call to address the problem led to a score of −1.0.

The Michel bill, too, recognized the problem and required that all antifraud provisions contain adequate procedures to protect individuals' privacy. All patient-specific information would have to be protected. The bill otherwise offered little, but on the other hand, the laissez-faire approach of Michel means that a universal, standardized data system would not be created. The looseness of Michel reflects the looseness of the current situation, in which employers, patients, and insurers develop their own systems and exercise choice. Thus the Michel approach represented the status quo plus somewhat greater privacy protection. The bill had no sanctions, and it did not address the privacy issues raised by large databases, but neither does the status quo. It thus earned a 1.0.

To sum up, the average scores for benchmark 8 are as follows:

McDermott/Wellstone	1.5
Clinton	3.1
Cooper	1.6
Michel	1.4

Benchmark 9: Comparability

Health care, however necessary, is not the only important social good. Health care reform should produce a mechanism that helps society to determine the relative worth of health care compared to all other goods and services. Consequently, this benchmark has only one criterion—the presence of a comprehensive budget for health care spending that would facilitate such comparisons.

Because it would establish a national budget for all health care spending, the single-payer approach provides the critical element needed for comparability. The McDermott/Wellstone bill required each state to have a similar type of budget. No budget was to rise faster than the gross national product, a stipulation that explicitly addresses comparability and the steady hijacking of funds from other parts of society over the past fifty years. Most health care facilities would also have had global budgets. This bill received a score of 5.0 on this benchmark.

The heavily managed competition approach of the Clinton plan is much more helpful than present practices, but less helpful than a single-payer approach, in determining how much of the social and national income is and should be spent on health care. States would monitor the financial status of the health plans and release this information to the public. The corporate alliances would perform similar monitoring activities. The very existence of the alliances would mean that budgets would be known and assembled under one body. Regional alliances would report to the states. Corporate alliances would report to the Secretary of Labor. Each could produce a comprehensive budget for their area or population, except for out-of-pocket expenditures. However, the system is not set up to deliberate about the relative worth of spending more money for health care compared to food stamps or building an information superhighway. The debate around the premium caps would provide a mechanism for public discussion comparing health care expenditures to other goods, but the premium caps would not include all health care expenditures. They also could not be enforced like global budgets. We scored it at 3.0.

Neither the Cooper nor Michel bills had any mechanism that would assure comparability, either in the form of global budgets or premium caps. Consequently, they both received a zero score on this benchmark. Much more thought needs to go into how market-based reforms can enable a nation to keep health care from appropriating funds from other social programs and to decide what the balance of funds should be among them.

In sum, the scores for benchmark 9 were as follows:

McDermott/Wellstone	5.0
Clinton	3.0
Cooper	0.0
Michel	0.0

Benchmark 10: Degree of Consumer Choice

Choice is a vital part of a fair health care system, though it must take place in a just context. The preceding benchmarks frame out that context. Choice is not fair if it is increased for some and decreased for others. Choice is not fair if some people have greater access than others (benchmarks 1 and 2) or if some have more benefits than others (benchmark 3) or if some have to pay disproportionately more than others (benchmarks 4 and 5). If a system gets poor value for its money (benchmarks 6 and 7), choice is limited for everyone. This is what has happened over the past decade. Public accountability (benchmark 8) is also a part of fair choice. It is discriminatory if some people have more information than others or managers covertly restrict choice.

In considering reform proposals, two issues stand out. The first is the danger that restructuring American health care into large managed care corporations (an approach not used by any of the countries that have provided ready access to good care and yet held costs steady over the past twenty years) will greatly reduce people's choices and replace them with the priorities of insurance companies, system executives, and investors. Their priorities are unlikely to emphasize distributive and social justice.

The second danger is that any reform, but especially reforms that put people into vertically integrated managed care systems, will medicalize American health care more than it is today (Caplan and Scarpaci 1989). We are referring to the fact that over one-third of Americans today use one or more therapists who are not physicians but who provide other kinds of treatment (Eisenberg et al. 1993). In 1990, Americans made over 400 million visits to alternative health care practitioners, more than the number of visits to all the nation's primary-care physicians. More than half of these patients first sought treatment within the biomedical paradigm and found it wanting. These patients spent about as much of their own money for alternative health care treatments as was spent by patients out of pocket for all hospitalizations.

If health care is organized into managed care systems with physicians as gatekeepers, it is likely that this large and growing sector of complementary medicine and healing would be excluded. Chiropractors, whose services are now widely insured, and to a lesser extent acupuncturists, could be shut out by unsympathetic gatekeepers (Caplan 1988). Alternate healing systems indigenous to Mexicans, Central Americans, Caribbeans, Indians, and Asians would remain outside managed care systems, even though they seem particularly apt for the chronic disorders and dysfunctions that characterize an aging population. Use of alternate systems reflects the ethnic and religious diversity of the United States. It also reflects the success of biomedicine in curing acute problems so that people are left with chronic ones. The criteria for including or excluding them in a fair health care system should be the same as for biomedicine: need and efficacy. For example, a three-year randomized trial comparing chiropractic with biomedical treatment of low back pain concluded that chiropractic treatment was more effective in reducing pain short and long term (Meade et al. 1990).

Fair health care reforms should not unduly restrict people's choice of any health practice or treatment, as long as it meets a clear need and is effective. Criteria for this benchmark concern the degree to which people can make full informed choices of their primary-care practitioners, of their medical specialists, of other licensed health care providers, and of the procedures any of them wish to undertake.

Choice of Primary-care Provider

The single-payer approach of the McDermott/Wellstone proposal allows eligible residents to choose any licensed primary-care provider. It keeps service in the private sector and uses the fee-schedule approach to allow all licensed practitioners to participate. It poses no financial or organizational barriers to care, and a universal data system would provide people with good information for weighing the options they have. For these reasons, this design earned a perfect score of 5.0.

Managed competition approaches to reform are designed to limit choice as a way to control costs. The heavily managed approach represented by Clinton was more open, because it required each health alliance to offer a fee-for-service option, which would include all the region's medical doctors and have no gatekeeper. This option, however, would probably be the most expensive, so that its degree of choice would be available primarily to affluent consumers, and its overall size would shrink over time. All other plans would be various forms of managed care. People could choose their plan and their primary-care doctors within the plan. This seems satisfactory except when the choice of primary-care provider is linked with choices among specialists so that people with serious medical problems who primarily choose the plan for its specialists or facilities may find that the primary-care doctor they like belongs to another plan.

A plan's executives may also drop some primary-care groups and sign on others, leaving the patients of a given group with a forced nonchoice. They would have to leave the entire plan and join one where their primary-care provider has a contract, or stay and settle for a different primary-care provider. One might call this "free chunky choice"; a person is free to choose within the managed care chunks assembled by investors, insurers, and managers. Chunky choice will also be economically biased, because plans can vary their premiums and co-payments so that the more costly plans offer more choice. Medicaid beneficiaries would be limited to the least costly plan, and many working-class Americans would probably feel equally restricted. Thus, while reforms based on competition between large managed care systems would reverse the present trajectory of less consumer choice, they earned a score of 3.5 rather than higher.

Under the version of lightly managed competition represented by the Cooper bill, all eligible individuals and small businesses would receive standardized information about each plan in the HPPC and then chose one. Within a plan they could choose their primary-care provider and could change once a year. The reforms also increased the supply of primary-care providers.

These reforms might offer some individuals slightly more choice of their primary-care provider than they have now, but they do not stop the present trajectory of decreasing consumer choice. As in the Clinton approach, health care plans could limit enrollment for reasons of financial insolvency or capacity limitations as they enrolled people on a first-come–first-served basis. Plans would have a greater range of premiums and co-pays than under the Clinton type of approach and therefore would be more economically discriminatory. The gap between the insured and the uninsured would remain quite large, and reductions in Medicare reimbursements could make it more difficult for beneficiaries to find primary-care providers. On balance, these reforms might result in a slight improvement of the current primary-care delivery system, and receive a score of 1.0.

The market-based Michel bill had similar features and limitations about choice as the Cooper bill. However, health insurance coverage would be less universal in Michel, thus restricting choice for the less affluent. The selective marketing and managing of for-profit insurance and service companies would exacerbate this problem. Those receiving medical assistance would be treated in the most restrictive ways. They could be required to enroll in a particular health plan or primary-care management company. A state could also narrow the period in which enrollees could leave a plan without due cause. The bill also required cost sharing for all services, except those related to prevention. If a state health plan (for the poor) has primary-care case management, it must ensure that all recipients have "reasonable choice" among the case managers. However, this term is not defined and applies only to case managers, not primary-care providers. On the more positive side, the Michel bill increased access to community and migrant health centers. These measures earned a 0.5 score on choice of primary-care provider.

Choice of Specialists

With respect to medical specialists, the single-payer approach of the McDermott/Wellstone bill would allow consumers to choose specialists or to belong to a managed care network and have their choices limited. The bill restored a free-choice system and therefore received a perfect score of 5.0.

Under the Clinton bill, managed care enrollees would be subject to the recommendations of their gatekeeping primary-care providers and the contractual choices of the plan's executives. They could go outside the network for specialty care but would have to pay more for these services. Medicare beneficiaries would continue to choose their own doctors. As noted above, each alliance would offer a fee-for-service plan, but it would be more expensive. Some special provisions would be made for the disabled, especially the severely disabled.

These reforms concerning medical specialists would significantly reduce specialty choice over current arrangements, especially for middle-class and working-class patients. The differences in how various plans configure specialty services and whom they choose are much greater than in primary care, because the differences in quality and consequences are greater in subspecialty fields and the stakes are higher among patients with serious problems. The far greater degree of control by insurance companies and other corporations that run managed care systems over rules, protocols, and their implementation on a case-by-case basis will most likely reduce access to costly subspecialty services.

Using a reform design that depends on managed care companies to restrict access poses inherent dangers to fair treatment. Co-payments in one form or another aggravate these problems. Alliances may have spotty or no cross-alliance agreements for using subspecialists outside their region. Those who could afford the fee-for-service option would escape these difficulties, but their ability to do so would be based solely on their income. Given how little evidence exists that competition between managed care systems actually saves money, these restrictions on choice seem unjustified. But counterbalancing all these concerns would be that the 36 to 40 million people who now have no choice would get limited choice. A score of −1.5 reflects this balance between more choice than none for some and less choice than now for most.

The lightly managed competition represented by the Cooper bill would drive most people into managed care, with all the concomitant problems already discussed. Cost sharing for all but preventive services and higher costs for out-of-network providers would be two more significant financial barriers reducing choice to see specialists. Class bias would also be greater than under the Clinton arrangements, with no guaranteed coverage for the uninsured to counterbalance these problems. Lower Medicare reimbursements would make it more difficult for beneficiaries to utilize medical specialists. These reforms would significantly worsen the present (1994) situation for the insured and reduce the uninsured by about half. We rated them a −3.5 based on 1993 practices. As more and more people and providers move into large managed care corporations, this score would go down because the status quo would become like Cooper's proposal.

The market-based approach represented by the Michel bill would allow still more cost sharing for most specialty care and more balance billing. It would also allow health plans (mostly managed) to charge their enrollees extra whenever they go outside the network for nonemergency care. However, the Michel approach would keep patterns closer to the status quo. More small-scale, clinically managed practices could continue under the loose provisions. On balance, we gave these reforms a −1.0 as slightly worse than current practices in 1993. As managed care systems become more prevalent, this score would fall towards −3.5.

Choice of Other Health Care Providers

With respect to other licensed health care providers, the McDermott/ Wellstone single-payer proposal allowed all licensed practitioners to be chosen by patients and therefore received a score of 5.0.

The Clinton proposal also allowed all licensed health providers to participate, but only as determined by managed care plans run by investors and insurers. The proposed National Health Board might have a biomedical bias in its decisions on needed and effective therapies. For these reasons, we gave the Clinton bill a −2.0 for reducing choice of alternate health care providers that existed in 1993. The Cooper bill had the same structural obstacles to choosing alternate providers and therefore received a −2.0 as well.

The Michel bill would also lead to managed care systems and decisions about what services are deemed "medically necessary" but with more looseness in the market structure and more room for coverage of alternate practices. We therefore scored it −1.0, as somewhat more restrictive towards coverage practices like chiropractic than now.

Choice of Procedure

Increasingly today, managed care systems restrict choice of procedure in various ways. They may state in their policy that certain procedures are not covered, in which case the restriction is at least fairly applied to all subscribers. But reports are coming in about hidden forms of reduced choice of procedures, such as by limiting the kinds and number of facilities and clinical teams in the system. Beside using strategies of inconvenience, some plans may tell therapists to keep the number of sessions below the number promised in the policy. For these reasons, choice of procedure has become distinct from choice of provider.

The relative fairness of the four bills concerning this issue is easy to score. The single-payer approach of McDermott and Wellstone would eliminate the growing restrictions on choice of procedure that now appear to be taking place, because the design leaves such matters up to individual providers. It therefore warranted a score of 5.0. The heavily managed competition approach of the Clinton bill would hasten such trends and leave plenty of room for managed care plans to carry out indirect if not direct restrictions. It therefore received a score of −3.0. The Cooper approach to lightly managed competition would also bolster managed care systems and received a score of −3.0 as well. The unmanaged approach of Michel would keep choice of procedure quite close to the present mixture of multiple arrangements and therefore had to receive a zero for not making this problem much better or worse than it is now.

The total average scores for this benchmark are:

McDermott/Wellstone	5.0
Clinton	−0.8
Cooper	−1.9
Michel	−0.4

Discussion

The overall scores for the four reform bills are summarized in tables 5–3 and 5–4. Only the single payer proposal reached our standard of 4.0 or better to make the American health care system about as fair as health care in other countries. But the important point is that the other three could have been much more fair. Only the single-payer proposal, with a grade of B (or 82 percent), comes close to our standard of 80 percent or better (4.0 or better), which is the score needed to make the American health care system about as fair as the systems in other countries. A heavily managed approach like the Clinton plan would make the American health care system notably more fair than now but still not as fair as other systems. Our benchmarks and criterion for each pinpoint just how. For example, Clinton's specific scores ranged from +5.0 to −3.0. This policy tool points to just which areas need more attention.

The significant point, however, is that the proposals that failed could have been much more fair. Any kind of delivery system can get fours and fives on how the money is collected (benchmarks 1 through 5). Likewise, any kind of delivery system would want high scores on benchmarks 6, 7, and 10. Enthoven's careful design of managed competition, which is the inspiration for nearly all proposals of this kind, would get high marks for fairness, because he gives so much attention to sources of unfairness and bias in health care markets. There is no reason why any proposal should not address issues of fairness fully.

Conclusion

The benchmarks of fairness take a general position about values, philosophy, and the just society, and translate them into ten specific benchmarks and thirty-one detailed criteria that provide a moral framework for anyone doing health care reform. Citizen groups, state legislators and managers, business health coalitions, federal legislative and executive committees, and others can now include fairness in their discussions. The detailed explanations of the benchmarks' application to a familiar spectrum of reform proposals give readers a richly textured model of how we think about provisions in a bill and their relationships to each other. Time and again we found that one provision was compromised or undermined by another. Or it applied to only one group or program. The amount of vagueness and promissory language would only warm the heart of a politician. Entire critical areas, like public accountability, were largely ignored.

Our actual scoring system is informal and imperfect. We hope that more

Table 5-3 Benchmarks of Fairness for United States Health Care Reform Proposals (Benchmarks 6–10)

	Public Financing/ Private Practice McDermott/ (Wellstone)	Heavily Regulated Market Approach (Clinton)	Moderately Regulated Market Approach (Cooper)	Least Regulated/ Free Market Approach (Michel)
Benchmark 6: *Value For Money—Clinical Efficacy*				
Emphasis on Primary Care	2.0	4.5	4.0	1.0
Emphasis on Public Health and Prevention	1.5	2.5	2.0	1.0
Systematic Assessment of Outcomes	4.5	3.5	2.5	2.0
Minimizing Overutilization and Underutilization	4.0	4.0	3.5	2.0
Average Score for Benchmark 6	3.0	3.6	3.0	1.5
Benchmark 7: *Value For Money—Financial Efficacy*				
Minimizing Administrative Overhead	5.0	3.0	2.5	2.0
Tough Contractual Bargaining	5.0	3.5	0.0	0.0
Minimizing Cost Shifting	5.0	3.0	2.0	0.0
Anti–Fraud and Abuse Measures	3.0	3.5	2.0	3.5
Average Score for Benchmark 7	4.5	3.3	1.6	1.4
Benchmark 8: *Public Accountability*				
Explicit Public Procedures for Evaluation	4.0	4.5	3.0	2.5
Explicit Democratic Procedures for Resource Allocation	2.0	2.0	0.5	0.0
Fair Grievance Procedures	1.0	5.0	4.0	2.0
Adequate Privacy Protection	−1.0	1.0	−1.0	1.0
Average Score for Benchmark 8	1.5	3.1	1.6	1.4
Benchmark 9: *Comparability*	5.0	3.0	0.0	0.0
Benchmark 10: *Degree of Consumer Choice*				
Choice of Primary-Care Provider	5.0	3.5	1.0	0.5
Choice of Specialists	5.0	−1.5	−3.5	−1.0
Choice of Other Health Care Providers	5.0	−2.0	−2.0	−1.0
Choice of Procedure	5.0	−3.0	−3.0	0.0
Average Score for Benchmark 10	5.0	−0.8	−1.9	−0.4

Explanation of Scores: Reform proposals were judged according to how much they would likely increase or decrease the fairness of the U.S. health care system. A score of zero represents no change from the status quo of 1994. Scores range from −5.0 to +5.0.

Table 5-4 Benchmarks of Fairness for United States Health Care Reform Proposals

	Public Financing/ Private Practice McDermott/(Wellstone)	Heavily Regulated Market Approach (Clinton)	Moderately Regulated Market Approach (Cooper)	Least Regulated Free Market Approach (Michel)
Benchmark 1:				
Universal Access—Coverage and Participation				
Mandatory Coverage and Participation	4.5	4.0	1.5	0.5
Prompt Phase-in	4.5	4.0	2.0	1.5
Portability	5.0	4.0	2.0	1.5
Average Score for Benchmark 1	4.7	4.0	1.8	1.2
Benchmark 2:				
Minimizing Nonfinancial Barriers				
Minimizing Maldistributions	5.0	4.5	0.5	0.5
Reform of Health Professional Education	4.0	4.0	4.0	0.0
Minimizing Language, Culture, Class Barriers	2.0	3.0	0.0	0.0
Minimizing Educational and Informational Barriers	2.0	4.5	3.5	3.0
Average Score for Benchmark 2	3.3	4.0	2.0	0.9
Benchmark 3:				
Comprehensive and Uniform Benefits				
Comprehensiveness	4.5	3.5	1.5	0.0
Reduced Tiering and Uniform Quality	3.0	2.5	1.5	0.0
Benefits Not Dependent on Savings	5.0	4.0	0.0	0.0
Average Score for Benchmark 3	4.2	3.3	1.0	0.0

Table 5-4 Benchmarks of Fairness for United States Health Care Reform Proposals (Continued)

	Public Financing/ Private Practice McDermott/(Wellstone)	Heavily Regulated Market Approach (Clinton)	Moderately Regulated Market Approach (Cooper)	Least Regulated Free Market Approach (Michel)
Benchmark 4: *Equitable Financing—Community-rated Contributions*				
True Community-rated Premiums	5.0	3.5	2.0	1.5
Minimum Discrimination via Cash Payments	5.0	1.5	0.5	0.0
Average Score for Benchmark 4	5.0	2.5	1.3	0.8
Benchmark 5: *Equitable Financing—By Ability to Pay*				
Equitable Financing—By Ability to Pay	5.0	2.0	1.0	0.0
Benchmark 6: *Value For Money—Clinical Efficacy*				
Emphasis on Primary Care	2.0	4.5	4.0	1.0
Emphasis on Public Health and Prevention	1.5	2.5	2.0	1.0
Systematic Assessment of Outcomes	4.5	3.5	2.5	2.0
Minimizing Overutilization and Underutilization	4.0	4.0	3.5	2.0
Average Score for Benchmark 6	3.0	3.6	3.0	1.5
Benchmark 7: *Value For Money—Financial Efficacy*				
Minimizing Administrative Overhead	5.0	3.0	2.5	2.0
Tough Contractual Bargaining	5.0	3.5	0.0	0.0
Minimizing Cost Shifting	5.0	3.0	2.0	0.0
Anti–Fraud and Abuse Measures	3.0	3.5	2.0	3.5
Average Score for Benchmark 7	4.5	3.3	1.6	1.4

Table 5-4 (Continued)

	Public Financing/ Private Practice McDermott/(Wellstone)	Heavily Regulated Market Approach (Clinton)	Moderately Regulated Market Approach (Cooper)	Least Regulated Free Market Approach (Michel)
Benchmark 8: *Public Accountability*				
Explicit Public Procedures for Evaluation	4.0	4.5	3.0	2.5
Explicit Democratic Procedures for Resource Allocation	2.0	2.0	0.5	0.0
Fair Grievance Procedures	1.0	5.0	4.0	2.0
Adequate Privacy Protection	−1.0	1.0	−1.0	1.0
Average Score for Benchmark 8	1.5	3.1	1.6	1.4
Benchmark 9: *Comparability*	5.0	3.0	0.0	0.0
Benchmark 10: *Degree of Consumer Choice*				
Choice of Primary-Care Provider	5.0	3.5	1.0	0.5
Choice of Specialists	5.0	−1.5	−3.5	−1.0
Choice of Other Health Care Providers	5.0	−2.0	−2.0	−1.0
Choice of Procedure	5.0	−3.0	−3.0	0.0
Average Score for Benchmark 10	5.0	−0.8	−1.9	−0.4
TOTAL: Average Score Across All Benchmarks	4.1	2.8	1.1	0.7

Explanation of Scores: Reform proposals were judged according to how much they would increase or decrease the fairness of the U.S. Health Care System. A score of zero represents no change from the status quo of 1994. Scores range from −5.0 to +5.0.

specific approaches to scoring are developed. A given group may wish to alter the criteria for a given benchmark or add a benchmark. They may have the resources to apply the criteria in a more comparative and rigorous way than was possible with this first effort. We urge further development of what we have been able to do.

From a substantive point of view, the current American system is much more unfair than any other health care system in the first world. American health care may be supreme in the world at its best, but it is quite uneven and discriminatory. As detailed in the development of the benchmarks and their application, forms of unfairness are found well beyond the problem of the uninsured.

6

Reorganization or Reform?
The Fairness of Current Trends

In August 1994, when the 103rd Congress abandoned any attempt to legislate national health care reform, we might have expected all talk about reform to cease, at least until some later Congress returned to the question. That has not happened (White 1994). Of course, some of the continued talk of reform was prompted by the belief that the states would pick up where the federal government had left off (Pear 1994). But the state reform initiatives that were passed in recent years have largely been put on hold, and some states are threatening to rescind them (Freudenheim 1995b). It is striking, then, given the failure of both federal and state reform efforts, to hear policy experts, politicians, and the media speak so assertively about ongoing "reform," even "dramatic" and "accelerating reform."

Some say that the market, unaided by government, is accomplishing what the government could not do (Anders and Stout, 1994). At the same time, although much of the change is market driven, the government is not completely inactive. Instead of legislating comprehensive or even incremental insurance coverage reform, Congress and President Clinton both propose major cuts or reductions in the rate of increases in the budgets for Medicare and Medicaid ("Democrats, GOP Trade Charges over Medicare" 1995). Some of the budget proposals are coupled with proposals to push many people on both forms of public insurance into managed care arrangements. The irony of these developments is that Harry and Louise, the middle Americans who complained in television ads that "big government" and the Clinton plan were the major threats to their choice of doctor and the quality of their care, would now have to proclaim (if anyone would pay them) that it is smaller government (budget cuts) and private managed care systems that are reducing choice, quality, and even coverage.

Is it abuse of language—Orwellian doublespeak—to call what is now happening in the health care system "reform"? We originally planned to call this chapter "Reorganization without Reform." We considered that "reform" indicated some intentional effort to achieve socially positive goals, such as assuring people access to needed health care or increasing value for money in the health care system. The market driven changes we are undergoing might or might not reduce health care costs, but they seemed unplanned—or is the invisible hand a planner?—and not necessarily directed at social improvement. It seemed misleading to label all change "reform."

We realized, however, that deeper political controversies underlay some of our semantic concerns. We wanted to reserve the "good" or "positive" word "reform" for government initiated efforts and the neutral word "reorganization" for nongovernmental, market-induced—seemingly unplanned—changes. But this usage ignores how much planning, albeit not government planning, is involved in these changes. It also ignores how some social improvement, specifically an increase in value for money or at least a reduction in costs to employers and government, is intended by those seeking to expand the use of managed care arrangements. The real question that concerns us in this chapter is not whether the word "reform" is being abused, but a more substantive matter, Are the market-driven changes now taking place fair?

The benchmarks of fairness can help us to understand how fair the current trends in our system are, whether those trends are market driven or government initiated. In the previous two chapters, we used the benchmarks to assess the fairness of types of health care reform proposals. In this chapter, we apply them to the consequences of passing none of these proposals. This legislative inaction left the existing and rapidly changing health care system in place, a system whose rate of change may have been accelerated by the very talk of reform. How do the changes taking place affect the fairness of the system? This chapter is designed to help answer this question.

We begin with a brief description of six major trends in American health care today. This description of current trends is crucial to the application of the benchmarks, since the benchmarks involve important empirical assumptions and their application focuses on the likely effects of organizational changes in American health care. Because our health care system is changing so quickly, our description is brief and unavoidably incomplete. We cannot specify all the causes or consequences of the six trends. This limitation necessarily makes our application of the benchmarks tentative and provisional.

In applying the benchmarks to our task, we take the summer of 1994 as a baseline. We also ignore ongoing speculation about further legislative changes and concentrate on the trends we describe. Our central question is this: Is the system being made more or less fair along each of the dimensions captured by the benchmarks? If the current trends are producing no significant change relative to our baseline for a given criterion, then a score of zero is given (on a scale from −5.0 to +5.0). As we noted in Chapter 2, a score of zero in this chapter means something different from a zero in Chapters 4 and 5. In chapters 4 and 5 a zero meant that the plan being assessed *proposed no change in the design of the system* on the dimension captured by the criterion being scored. A zero in chapter 4 or 5 is compatible with the trends actually at work in the unreformed system making it more or less fair over time. Since in this chapter we are examining the effects of the current trends over time, there is no direct comparability between a zero in this chapter and a zero in chapter 4 or 5. We bring this point out in the discussion when we occasionally compare scores in this chapter with the results of the Michel plan, which attempted the least governmental reform.

Some other modifications in the criteria are needed because of the change in our question from earlier chapters. For example, the criterion referring to the phase-in of reform now does not apply. In many cases where we assign a score, we must simply weigh conflicting trends against each other and average them. The reader is cautioned here (as earlier) not to take the numbers too seriously and to read them as indicating qualitative shifts and relative positions, not as assigning a real metric to changes.

Six Major Health Care Trends

To assess the fairness of ongoing changes in the health care system, we needed an overview of the types of changes taking place. To construct that overview, we conducted a literature review, did a content analysis on leading newspaper and magazine coverage, and conducted a telephone survey of officers of business and trade groups, unions, professional associations, and policy centers.* Based on our analysis of these sources of information, we chose to focus on these six trends:

* The content analysis concentrated on the nation's leading newspapers and magazines, such as *The New York Times*, *The Wall Street Journal*, *The Washington Post*, *The Los Angeles Times*, *Newsweek*, and *Time*. The telephone survey involved asking these questions: What do you think are the three most important trends currently taking place in our health care system? And, what do you think their likely impact will be on access, cost, and quality of care? The questions were addressed to knowledgeable people at the following nineteen institutions and organizations:

Think Tanks:
American Enterprise Institute, The Rand Corporation, Brookings Institute, National Health Policy Forum.

Labor Unions:
American Federation of Labor-Congress of Industrial Organizations, American Federation of State County and Municipal Employees, Communications Workers of America.

1. cost cutting in government programs, both state and federal;
2. expansion of managed care;
3. corporatization of health care;
4. increasing numbers of uninsured and underinsured;
5. rising out-of-pocket expenditures;
6. ambulatory and community-based services displacing hospital care.

Because the American health care system is changing so rapidly, our simplified list of six major trends must be seen as but a snapshot of a complex, dynamic process. We ignore some changes and focus on those that have either greatly accelerated since our baseline, the summer of 1994, or that are relatively new but are likely to become more important over time. The trends involve changes that are themselves complex, intertwined, and sometimes even contradictory. Our assessment must be tentative, since much of the evidence for the trends is anecdotal or incomplete. Hard evidence and firm numbers will not be available for some time. Let us briefly describe each of these trends.

Cutting Government Costs

In November 1994, conservative Republicans, who promised balanced budgets and lower taxes, gained control of Congress, most state capitals, and many large municipal governments, such as New York City. Since then, the pressure to reduce government spending on health care has become much more focussed and more intense (Lueck 1995). At the federal level, Medicare and Medicaid, entitlements programs for the elderly and about half the poor, respectively, have been targeted for large spending cutbacks (Toner 1995). For example, House Republicans want to reduce Medicare spending by $282 billion over the next seven years. Senate Republicans look for $256 billion in Medicare savings. Since Medicare spending is approximately $178 billion in 1995, either of these cuts would prove substantial (Milhiser 1995). Some Democrats, including President Clinton, also support reductions in Medicare spending, although their projected savings are somewhat lower ("Democrats, GOP Trade Charges over Medicare" 1995). This drive to reduce government spending on Medicare will likely

---

Professional Organizations:
American Manufacturing Association, American Medical Association, American Psychological Association, Association of State and Territorial Health Officers, Physicians for National Health Program.

Business/Trade Groups:
Washington Business Group, Business Roundtable, Health Insurance Association of America, Employee Benefit Research Institute, National Association of Manufacturers, United States Chamber of Commerce.

Political Organizations:
National Governors' Association.

accelerate efforts to reduce payments to doctors and hospitals further, to raise out-of-pocket expenses, and to increase enrollments in managed care (Roberts 1993).

Medicaid is also a major target. House Republicans want to convert it to a block grant, cut its annual growth rate in half (from 8 percent to 4 percent), and turn it completely over to the states (Milhiser 1995). Medicaid is already one of the states' largest and fastest growing budget items, and many states are already cutting back on their Medicaid spending. For example, New Jersey recently announced a 20-percent cut in Medicaid reimbursements to hospitals (Sullivan 1994). Similarly, New York governor George Pataki wants to cut $1.2 billion from his Medicaid budget, the deepest cut in the state's history (Jones 1994).

Expanding Managed Care

Over the past year, the move to managed care has become a stampede (Schroeder 1994:14). Nationally, nearly 60 million people currently belong to Health Maintenance Organizations (HMOs)—a record 15.8 percent increase over 1994 (Health Insurance Association of America 1995). An additional 75 million belong to Preferred Provider Organizations (PPOs). Altogether, approximately one-half of the nation's population is currently enrolled in some form of managed care (Health Insurance Association of America 1995). Managed care enrollments do vary greatly by state, however. This means the effects of current changes are being felt more in some states than others.

The private sector is leading the stampede. Currently, approximately 58 percent of employees of small businesses (10–499 employees) are enrolled in managed care. The comparable figure for large businesses (five hundred or more employees) is 66 percent ("How Managed Care Is Restructuring the Health Care Industry" 1995). In total, about 50 percent of all full-time workers are currently enrolled in some type of managed care plan (Schroeder 1994:14).

The public sector is clearly behind but trying to catch up. Currently, only about 9 percent of Medicare and 23 percent of Medicaid beneficiaries are enrolled in managed care. ("How Managed Care Is Restructuring the Health Care Industry" 1995). By the end of the decade, around 70 percent of all these people will likely be enrolled in some form of managed care (Gorski 1995). Most of this growth will be among the Medicaid population (Winslow 1995a). Many elderly seem resistant about participating and most politicians are reluctant to force them (Lewis 1995). However, states are increasingly requiring their Medicaid populations to join managed care plans (*Medicaid: States Turn To Managed Care* 1993). Last year, forty-five states and the District of Columbia had Medicaid managed care plans, and over half of them were mandatory (Schroeder 1994:14).

In at least three important ways, managed care is dramatically changing American health care. First, the spread of capitated payments and the concomitant decline of fee-for-service are radically restructuring risk. Risk is being shifted from insurance companies to doctors and hospitals. As we will see shortly, this shift fundamentally changes all sorts of incentives about who to insure and the type and quality of services they receive (Pallarito 1994). Second, the distinction between insurance and health care delivery is being blurred, even eliminated. More specifically, managed care combines these two activities into one organization. Some managed care organizations are set up and run by an insurance company. Others are sponsored by health care providers, such as physicians or hospitals (Goldstein and Baker 1995). In the former, the insurer contracts for the delivery of services. In the latter, the deliverers are also the insurers. Finally, managed care is accelerating an information revolution in American medicine. Managed care requires large integrated data systems for patient tracking, physician profiling and enrollee education (Light 1994e). Unfortunately managed care organizations do not appear to be using data systems that can be integrated across plans, so comparative outcomes research and epidemiological studies cannot be done.

Corporatization of Health Care

The corporatization of American medicine involves both the amalgamation of professional practices into large, corporate units and their expansion into the public sector. The priorities of investors increasingly shape the organization of health care, clinical decisions, and the market itself. The fastest growing form of managed care, to name one instance, is the for-profit HMO or PPO (Schroeder 1994), and for-profit hospitals are increasingly dominating their markets (De Lafuente 1994).

Mergers, takeovers, and partnerships among hospitals, pharmaceutical, and managed care companies are occurring at record levels. For example, in 1994, there were forty-three announced or completed acquisitions and mergers valued at $200 million or more each. The total value of these consolidations was nearly $60 billion, a record. In 1993, there were only twenty-one such transactions, with a combined value of about $24 billion "Consolidation Mania" 1995).

More Uninsured, More Underinsured

The fourth trend, an increase in the number of uninsured and the thinning out of coverage among those with insurance, is not new. Between 1987 and 1993, the net number of uninsured increased by over a million a year, jumping from 31 to 39 million. During the past year and a half, approximately two to three million more Americans have become uninsured, bring-ing the total to between 41 and 43 million people (Weiner 1994:12; Bradsher 1995). The principal causes lie in both the public and private sectors. In the public sector two principal problems are Medicaid cutbacks and the privatization of government services. In the private sector, the biggest problem is the shrinkage of employer-based health insurance, espe-cially for retirees and small-business employees (Employee Benefit Re-search Institute 1994). Between 1988 and 1994, over four million people under the age of 65 lost employer-sponsored health insurance (Holahan, Winterbottom, and Rojan 1995).

Insured employees are having their coverage destabilized and reduced in several ways: by capping how much will be paid for procedures, by increas-ing co-payments, and by managed plans that use protocols to decide what treatments are allowed. Private insurers continue to use preexisting exclu-sions and waiting periods to limit coverage (Light 1994a). They are also limiting benefits in the treatment of mental illness, drug addictions, and childbirth. For example, many HMOs now require women to leave the hospital within twenty-four hours after giving birth. This restriction has caused an uproar, especially in New Jersey where it was recently outlawed (Reinhardt 1995b). Increasing numbers of small employers, exempted from state mandates, are also offering "thinner" coverage (Fisher 1995). In the public sector, Medicaid and Medicare coverage are also being trimmed (Hudson 1995).

Patients Pay More

The fifth trend, also not new, is escalating out-of-pocket expenditures. This trend is evident in both the public and private sectors. For example, Medi-care premiums, co-payments, and deductibles are steadily going up. The elderly now pay about 28 percent of the cost of their care out of pocket. This represents a 50-percent increase, as a share of their income, compared to when Medicare started (Binstock 1994). Another round of increases is expected soon (Rosenbaum 1995). In the private sector, workers are also paying more for their health care. This cost shifting usually takes the form of higher premium payments, deductibles, and coinsurance rates. For exam-ple, many state employees are being asked to pay part of their premiums. In unmanaged care, co-payments and deductibles are increasing rapidly, a main part of the reason many are joining managed care plans.

Dehospitalization

The final trend is the displacement of hospital care by ambulatory and community-based services. Of course, hospital occupancy rates and average lengths of stay have been declining for over a decade (Coile 1990). However, managed care and new medical technologies have significantly accelerated the growth of outpatient services, especially home care, which is the fastest growing part of U.S. health care (Fusco 1994). In 1982, outpatient services accounted for 13 percent of all hospital revenues; now it accounts for 20 percent ("HHS Proposes Outpatient Prospective Payment" 1995).

This trend is most striking among teaching hospitals, Medicare recipients, and the mentally ill. For example, between 1994 and 1998, the number of inpatient days at major teaching hospitals is expected to fall by 24 percent, while outpatient procedures increase by 14 percent (Iglehart 1995a). With respect to Medicare, home care is its fastest growing component and half of all Medicare surgeries are now done on an outpatient basis ("HHS Proposes Outpatient Prospective Payment" 1995). Similarly, there has been a marked increase in outpatient psychiatry, much to the detriment of the psychiatric hospital (Fried 1995).

The trend toward outpatient care is important because of its implications for health care costs and the organization of delivery systems, the impetus it provides for the integration of hospitals with provider networks, and the opportunity this provides for the corporatization of health care.

Assessing the Fairness of Current Trends

We noted earlier that the question we asked in applying the benchmarks in this chapter is different from the question we asked in the previous two chapters, and so we have had to modify the meaning of our scale and adjust the criteria accordingly. The tentative nature of the scoring is forced by the complexity of current trends and the scarcity of hard data concerning them. Since our primary concern is to illustrate the process of analyzing the implications of these trends for judgments about fairness, the provisional nature of these scores should help encourage further debate and analysis rather than settle the issues addressed.

Benchmark 1: Universal Access—Coverage and Participation

This benchmark is scored on two criteria: (1) mandatory participation and universal coverage and (2) full portability and continuity of coverage. We have dropped the criterion used in previous chapters that referred to the speed of phase-in since it does not apply here.

Mandatory Coverage and Participation

Approximately two million people have lost their health insurance since the summer of 1994 (Hellander et al. 1995). The number of uninsured is expected to rise again this year (Eckholm 1994; Bradsher 1995). This continuing movement is important because it occurs during a period when the economy improved and unemployment decreased. Market forces have not worked to increase coverage with increased employment because of the trend we noted earlier, the reduction in coverage by many employers. Relying on the market seems, then, to involve "abandoning the idea . . . of universal access and universal coverage" (Kent 1995, p. 3), although it keeps concerns about cost containment alive (Tumulty 1994).

The forces are familiar ones, and we have commented on them earlier. For example, in an attempt to keep costs to employers down, medical underwriting is being used vigorously in small- and medium-size groups to avoid large categories of more costly people (Light 1992b). The privatization of public services by some states is worsening the access problem (Bell 1995). When states privatize their services, workers are no longer state employees and no longer part of a union. Consequently, even if they are rehired by the private employer, they have no health insurance. The loss of manufacturing jobs, which usually provide health insurance, and the greater use of "contingent workers" are causing similar access problems in the private sector (Hammonds 1994).

Overall, the nation seems farther away from universal access than it was in our baseline year (Freudenheim 1995b). Since the trends at work are gradual, and there is no markedly new force at work or indication of a rapid acceleration in the loss of coverage, we give this a score of -1.0. This score might seem too low, for in chapter 4 we roughly calibrated a score of 1.0 to a reduction in the uninsured of about 3 percent. But we wanted to signal a significant negative tendency that acts in the face of increasing employment and a growing economy. A much larger loss of coverage or indication of a new force at work would produce a higher negative score.

Portability

Had state insurance reforms replaced the failure of national reform, as some initially suggested would happen (Pear 1994), there might have been an improvement here. But, as we noted earlier, important state reforms under consideration or actually enacted prior to our baseline year have been put aside (Freudenheim 1995b). The New York state legislation to impose community rating in insurance and to improve portability by blocking exclusions for prior conditions has actually led many low-risk insurees to drop their coverage, thwarting the intended effect.

The influences that lead to less coverage, which we noted in discussion of the previous criterion, also negatively affect portability and continuity of coverage. Since we see no dramatic worsening of portability, and since we have no clear measures of decreased portability or continuity to compare to the estimates of increased numbers of uninsured, we score this criterion a modest negative score, -0.5.

The average score for benchmark 1 is -0.75. This score reflects the growing number of uninsured and the suspending of state insurance reforms passed or under consideration in our baseline year. It represents a slight decrease in the fairness of the existing health care system.

It is worth explaining briefly why the market-based Michel bill evaluated in chapter 4 received higher scores than the market-driven changes we assess here. We estimated in chapter 4 that the insurance reform incorporated in the Michel bill, prohibiting exclusions for high risk, would have increased coverage slightly. This and other reforms would have also positively improved portability. In chapter 4 we asked whether Michel's proposal improved the system relative to its design in the baseline year, and the answer was slightly positive. In this chapter, we ask whether the unreformed system is becoming fairer or not, given current trends. The answer is slightly negative. Had the Michel bill involved no improvement in the status quo, it would have received a zero, which is still different from the score in this chapter.

Benchmark 2: Universal Access—Minimizing Nonfinancial Barriers

The score for this benchmark is based on the degree to which changes in our health care system (1) minimize maldistributions of personnel, equipment, and facilities; (2) reform health education; (3) minimize language, cultural, and class barriers; and (4) minimize educational and informational barriers.

Minimizing Maldistributions

Our discussion of the trends suggests that forces are at work in both the public and private sectors that will redistribute resources over time. These forces include budget cutbacks in the public sector, the expansion of managed care in both sectors, and the corporatization of delivery systems in the private sector. The specific question posed by this criterion, however, is whether the redistribution that results improves the availability of services in underserved areas and decreases it in areas with excess services.

Evidence suggests that resources are actually flowing into more affluent areas while they are leaving chronically underserved areas, making the maldistribution worse. For example, many rural and urban hospitals are closing, downsizing, or teetering on the edge (Myers 1995). Large public hospitals in New York City, Washington, D.C., Boston, and Chicago are all in financial trouble (Watson 1995). Facing bankruptcy, Los Angeles County recently proposed closing County USC Medical Center, a large public hospital serving the poor and uninsured, the busiest hospital in the country (M. Davis 1995; Sack 1995). According to the president of the National Association of Public Hospitals, "elected officials are throwing up their hands and putting hospitals on the block, threatening to make substantial changes, or even close them" (Watson 1995, p. 1). In addition, large hospital chains are buying up community hospitals and closing vital services, such as obstetrics (Freudenheim 1995a). At the same time, suburban hospitals are "financially well off" and expanding (Stewart 1995). Similar reallocations are also taking place with medical equipment and personnel ("Scherer's Pact with Marquest" 1993). The absence of adequate primary-care personnel in many poor urban areas is likewise frustrating the effort to cut costs by using managed care arrangements for Medicaid patients (Fisher and Fein 1995).

Of course, given this country's excess hospital capacity, not every hospital closing represents a maldistribution of resources. Our chief concern is that this downsizing is being done without an overall plan and that there are inadequate safeguards to protect the most vulnerable.

On balance, the unfair resource allocations of the marketplace overshadow any distributional improvements that result from small-scale technological changes, such as the increased use of telemedicine (Busack 1994; Perednia 1995). Consequently, we score this criterion −1.0.

Reform of Health Professional Education

The expansion of capitated managed care is bolstering the demand for primary care, while reducing the demand for medical specialists (Meyer 1994; Rosenthal 1995). Because of this decline in the demand for specialty care, fewer students are choosing these specialties and more are retraining to deliver primary care (Rosenthal 1995). For example, the number of students applying for anesthesiology residencies is down 30 to 50 percent in 1994–5 (from a level producing a significant oversupply). Some residents are dropping out and starting over in other fields, such as family practice or emergency medicine (Anders 1995b). This shift in resources away from specialty care is a positive development in medical education because it realigns workforce training with health care needs.

Without a significant reallocation of training funds toward primary-care education, however, it is not clear just how strong this will be. The closing of public hospitals, where many residency programs are located ("Harvard Hospitals to Cut Residents" 1995), and future cutbacks in Medicare, an important funder of medical education, also raise concerns about the availability of training for primary care in underserved areas.

Since there is some definite movement toward decreasing specialty training, and only uncertainty about the availability of new primary-care training, we (tentatively) score this criterion +2.0. Remember that the market-based Michel bill received a score of zero, indicating it proposed keeping the status quo, but our analysis in this chapter suggests the unreformed system has some positive tendencies regarding this criterion.

Minimizing Language, Cultural, and Class Barriers

We do not see any tendency of the six trends to move the system one way or the other with regard to these barriers. Consequently, they receive a score of zero.

Minimizing Educational and Informational Barriers

Many managed care enrollees, especially Medicare HMO participants, do not adequately understand enrollment and appeal procedures, cost sharing, and service access (Winslow, 1993). As the managed care market expands, so too may this consumer ignorance. At the same time, many managed care organizations are educating enrollees about their particular health problems and how to take better care of themselves. We think these tendencies so far cancel each other and give a score of zero for this criterion.

The average score for this benchmark is 0.25, but understanding the reasoning behind each score, provisional as it must be, is more important than this uninformative number.

Benchmark 3: Comprehensive and Uniform Benefits

We have reduced the three criteria used for this benchmark in chapter 4 to two for our application in this chapter. First, all effective and needed services are to be made affordable and available, with no categorical exclusions of services, such as mental health or long-term care. Second, differences in the quality of services or providers, or tiering, are to be minimized. We eliminated the original third criterion, which required that the range of benefits not be dependent on "savings" generated elsewhere through reform, since it does not apply.

Comprehensiveness

There are several ways to reduce the comprehensiveness of benefits. Whole categories of services may be denied or services within them capped, without the limits taking into account the relative importance or effectiveness of those services. At this point, we have no definitive evidence of any specific increase or decrease in this practice with the advance of managed care or as a result of budget cuts in public programs. There is anecdotal evidence of some forms of this practice. For example, several managed care plans and other insurers in Massachusetts have refused to pay for certain kinds of neuropsychological evaluation, insisting that these previously covered services be paid for by school systems.

Another way of limiting comprehensiveness is by lowering the amount of services available for particular conditions. This may be done by restricting access to specialists capable of delivering those services or by developing practice guidelines or protocols that constrain how practitioners may treat patients or refer them for treatment by others. However, the mere fact of restriction is not itself grounds for a negative score on this criterion. The restrictions must mean that some needed and effective treatments are denied, not that they are replaced by other less expensive but reasonably effective or appropriate alternatives. Managed care organizations have been accused of denying services to people with chronic conditions, like mental illness, physical disabilities, AIDS, and drug addictions (Frank 1994). Other managed care organizations try to avoid these people in the first place (Osher and Christianson 1994).

At this point, we do not believe we have adequate information to assign a score to this criterion. We fear that threatened funding reductions to the Agency for Health Care Policy Research and the Office of Technology Assessment may make it much harder to find out the effects of managed care restrictions on treatments for certain types of patients.

Reduced Tiering and Uniform Quality

In our application of the benchmarks to reform proposals in Chapter 4, tiering was an important consideration because subsidies for low-income people would determine the type of managed care insurance they could buy, and there was a widespread concern that reform not replicate the existing tiering of Medicaid patients. The most important development concerning tiering is the "mainstreaming" of Medicaid recipients in some states into HMOs. Our understanding is that the managed care organizations into which Medicaid recipients are enrolled in these states must serve a wider patient population; they are not specifically set up for Medicaid recipients. To the degree that this trend develops, tiering will be significantly reduced. Tiering will also be constrained by the extent that Medicare recipients are also given incentives to enroll in managed care organizations. In New York, however, there is growing evidence that an inadequate supply of primary-care physicians and oversubscription of Medicaid recipients by some managed care organizations has led to strong complaints about inadequate access to treatment and has made many patients to seek emergency rooms without prior approval because they claim they cannot see their primary-care physicians (Fisher and Fein 1995).

Yet in the private sector there is also a contrary trend. More and more small employers are obtaining ERISA exemptions and avoiding all state-mandated benefits. These exemptions not only allow employers to provide less comprehensive benefits but further distinguish between health benefits covered by state mandates and those which are not (Darling 1995).

Current trends seem to be producing some conflicting effects on quality of care. Across the country, as hospitals, especially public hospitals, struggle to cut costs, registered nurses are being replaced by unlicensed nurse's aides and other types of "care associates" (Cowley, Miller, and Hager 1995). Referring to such substitutions, one doctor in a Nashville, Tennessee hospital stated "Some of the people I'm [now] relying on to be my eyes and ears have less training than the person running the slushy machine at 7-Eleven" (Cowley, Miller, and Hager 1995, p. 86). The University Community Hospital in Tampa, Florida, recently suggested that family members help with patient care (Gordon 1995). This deskilling of nurses, the largest group of hospital employees, threatens the quality of hospital care. Managed care organizations also try to substitute less expensive forms of providers for more highly credentialed providers. There is a lack, however, of controlled outcomes studies on the effects of these cost-saving measures, and there is a concern that managed care organizations may have a conflict of interest in carrying out those studies by themselves.

According to their supporters, managed care organizations screen providers carefully, employing only highly competent health care providers, and they closely monitor their performance. As a result, the quality of their care is excellent (Dubois and Blank 1995). In this way, managed care organizations are also creating a more uniform quality of care. In fact, a stream of studies over the past fifteen years documents that care for some problems in HMOs is superior to fee-for-service care. The new HMOs and rapidly expanding managed care corporations, however, may behave differently from the HMOs that saw themselves as having a mission to care for the "whole" patient. So far, the new managed care corporations appear to "save money" mainly by extracting sizable discounts from doctors and hospitals. As that source of profits is exhausted, some observers fear quality will decline (Nordgren 1995). Already, *among the sick*, those in managed care report less access and poorer care than those treated by independent providers (RWJ 1995).

There seems to be a slight trend toward less tiering, but most of it is the result of policies in the public sector to expand the use of managed care, not market forces themselves. Maldistributions of personnel may frustrate this trend. The evidence about quality is inconclusive, and much depends on whether the new entrants into managed care perform as well as the earlier HMOs. Overall, we score this criterion a +1.0. Since we did not score the criterion for comprehensiveness of benefits, and since the original third criterion does not apply, there is no computable average for this benchmark. For purposes of entry in the table at the end of this chapter, we list the benchmark score as +1.0*, where the asterisk indicates incomplete scoring.

Benchmark 4: Equitable Financing—Community-Rated Contributions

There are two criteria for this benchmark, the true community rating of premiums and minimum discrimination against the sick via out-of-pocket payments.

True Community-Rated Premiums

New York state mandated community rating of insurance, but it did so without any requirement for universal coverage. The result was predicted by many: numerous low-risk insurees dropped their coverage to avoid escalating premiums. Nationally, the trends in the system, however, continue to work against true community rating. To lower costs to small- and middle-sized employers, insurers continue to resort to medical underwriting and experience rating. The pressure to do so will grow as it becomes harder for managed care providers to decrease costs by securing even lower discounts from hospitals and other providers. We have already discussed the effects of this underwriting on insurance coverage for those at higher risk.

We have, however, no strong evidence that the use of experience rating is increasing significantly in the period since our baseline year. We signal our concern that the pressures against community rating are increasing by scoring this criterion a -0.5.

Minimum Discrimination via Cash Payments

The expansion of managed care has led to some reduction in out-of-pocket expenditures in the form of co-payments and deductibles. The prospect of pushing Medicare patients into managed care organizations would also expand this trend (Kongstvedt 1995). If there is significant "thinning" of benefit packages in new managed care plans, however, then out-of-pocket expenditures would be raised for those who need the reduced benefits. Furthermore, cash payments are multiplying for those not in managed care arrangements. For example, in the indemnity market, these increases take the form of service caps, higher deductibles, and longer waiting periods.

We see these trends as offsetting each other and score this criterion a zero.

For the benchmark as a whole, the average score is -0.25, which reflects no significant change in the fairness—or rather, the unfairness—of the system on this benchmark. For many people, our health care system makes expenditures for insurance and services depend to a consequential degree on levels of risk, violating the principle underlying this benchmark. The modest change under current trends must be judged against the quite general failure to fund health care without attention to degree of risk.

Benchmark 5: Equitable Financing—By Ability to Pay

This benchmark requires that all direct and indirect payments and out-of-pocket expenses are scaled to household budgets and one's ability to pay.

There are no federal or state initiatives that would provide subsidies to low-income individuals beyond those that existed in our baseline year. Nor are there any initiatives to scale indirect payments according to ability to pay. The trends in our system continue an already inequitable financing system, but they do not seem to make it better or worse than it already was in our baseline year. We score them a zero.

Benchmark 6: Value for Money—Clinical Efficacy

The first two criteria for this benchmark concern the advancement of primary care and the provision of public health and other forms of prevention. The second two criteria concern the systematic assessment of outcomes and the minimization of both over- and underutilization of services.

Emphasis on Primary Care and on Public Health and Prevention

The advance of managed care is giving primary care and clinical prevention a much needed boost (De Lafuente 1994b). Most managed care organizations employ a higher than average ratio of primary-care physicians and stress preventive services (Weiner 1994). Unfortunately, these advances are largely limited to managed care. Outside of managed care, there is no similar emphasis. For some, especially the uninsured, access to primary care may be declining (Weissman and Epstein 1994).

Still, the overall focus on primary care has improved since our baseline year, and we score the first criterion a +2.0. We note that the "market-based" Michel bill received a score of +1.0 for this criterion in chapter 4, which reflects the different uses of the benchmarks in the two chapters. The low positive score in chapter 4 was for specific but modest measures that the bill *proposed* to improve outpatient primary care, including funding for community and migrant health centers. In this chapter, we are judging how the expansion of managed care itself *actually* improves the primary care.

The story is quite different for the criterion that concerns public health and prevention. Increasing competition in the health care marketplace, coupled with governmental cutbacks, is squeezing our public health system (Lashof 1994). Public health expenditures are now less than 2 percent of total health care spending ("Finding More Money for the Core of Public Health" 1994). While many public health problems, from childhood diseases to AIDS, grow steadily worse, our public health infrastructure continues to deteriorate (Califano 1994). However, this deterioration is not new; public health in the United States has long been in "disarray" (Institute of Medicine 1988). Whether expanding managed care networks and a shrinking public sector are ultimately compatible with effective public health remains to be seen ("Public Health Threatened" 1995). We are also concerned with congressional proposals to cut environmental health protections and to further reduce funding for occupational health and safety enforcement. We thus provisionally score this criterion a −1.0.

Systematic Assessment of Outcomes and Minimizing Overutilization and Underutilization

Managed care organizations are creating large data systems and systematically assessing the outcomes of an extensive variety of clinical procedures. They are also developing protocols or practice guidelines for many of their procedures. There are now corporations emerging that conduct safety and efficacy analyses of new technologies and of the practice guidelines being developed by managed care organizations. This is proprietary information, however, and must be purchased by providers. Some forms of "outcomes research" are thus becoming more common and more widely used in the private sector. There is also some evidence that patient care is directly benefiting from these efforts (Crosson 1995). This type of medical care management is certainly a positive development.

Nevertheless, we have misgivings about the prospects for outcomes assessment in the current health care system. The Republican Congress has taken some steps to dramatically reduce funding for outcomes research, specifically targeting the Office of Technology Assessment and the Agency for Health Care Policy Research, which had funded much of the development of practice guidelines since 1989. Since outcomes assessment by managed care organizations is largely proprietary information, we know little about how it is conducted or what the results really mean. For example, managed care organizations with high turnover rates and short-term profit goals may be less interested in the long-term benefits of some practices. Reducing publicly funded studies that cut across health care plans is thus a serious loss.

Were it not for the threat to publicly funded outcomes research, we would score this criterion a +1.5, despite the shortcomings of leaving assessment to managed care organizations that have somewhat narrow interests. Our concerns about the public funding of this research cause us to reduce this score, at least provisionally, to a +0.5. If publicly funded outcomes assessment is sustained, we would raise this score.

There are conflicting trends and conflicting evidence about the minimization of both over- and underutilization. On the positive side, managed care organizations, through rigorous case management and clinical protocols, are significantly reducing the overutilization of medical services, especially hospital services (Light 1994e). All of the incentives of managed care and various forms of capitated reimbursement push in the direction of reducing utilization. The nonmanaged care sector has less capability of undertaking these sorts of measures.

But what can be said about avoiding underutilization of services? We face considerable anecdotal evidence and little in the way of solid studies. For example, growing numbers of mental health professionals and their patients are complaining that under managed care, therapy is inappropriately denied or truncated (Eckholm 1993:221–6). In fact, at least one state, Pennsylvania, is currently investigating the criminal denial of mental health care (Fried 1995).

In the hospital industry, capitated managed care and powerful insurers are driving down average lengths of stay. But, since the United States already has the world's shortest hospital stays, further reductions may be unwarranted. On the other hand, it could be that stays are unnecessarily long nearly everywhere else and they are still too long in the United States. Or, perhaps hospital stays are being safely shortened through an increase in the supply of outpatient services. In short, we know the pattern is changing, but we do not know the actual degree of underutilization. We suspect some of it is a good development, but some may constitute the denial of needed health care.

In addition, consolidations, closings, and cutbacks of public hospitals are making the situation even worse. For example, in New York's public hospitals, too few caesareans seem to be endangering the health of poor women and their babies (Fritsch and Baquet 1995). At a demonstration in Washington, D.C., in March 1995, nurses from across the country expressed similar apprehensions about their hospitals ("Nurses Protest Layoffs, Care Cuts" 1995).

Although much of the evidence concerning the underutilization of care is largely anecdotal, it can not be entirely dismissed ("Prognosis Not Clear on Affect of Nurse Cuts" 1995). It is after all, much more difficult to document the underutilization rather than the overutilization of a service. There is also some evidence, which we cited earlier, that patients who are already sick protest more about access and lack of treatment in managed care organizations than they do in other delivery contexts (RWJ 1995).

We score this criterion a +2.0 since there is stronger evidence of controls on overutilization than there is of extensive underutilization. But this score, like others in this chapter, is provisional since we lack important information.

Overall, this benchmark receives a score of +0.9. This appears to be a case in which the trends in the market-driven system would produce higher positive scores if the public sector upheld its commitments to outcomes research and the provision of public health. Political, not market, trends reduce the scores on this benchmark.

Benchmark 7: Value for Money—Financial Efficiency

The first two criteria for this benchmark require minimizing administrative overhead, such as unnecessary bureaucratic costs and excessive profits, and establishing tough bargaining between buyers and sellers. The third and fourth criteria require the minimization of cost shifting and adequate measures against fraud and abuse.

Minimizing Admininistrative Overhead

Managed care involves relatively high administrative costs. Between 13 and 20 percent of the health care budget under managed care is spent on administrative expenses, such as consultants, marketing, physician profiling, and patient monitoring (Light 1993b). For example, HMOs and PPOs in New Jersey have administrative costs of 14 to 20 percent. Traditional health plans in the state have administrative costs of around 4.5 percent. In other words, the typical HMO now spends about 83 percent of its revenue on medical care (Hilzenrath 1994). Included in the nonmedical expenditures are the high salaries of managers. In 1994, the seven largest for-profit HMOs paid their chief executives an average of $7 million in cash and stock (Freudenheim 1995c).

Administrative costs are also increasing for providers. They now spend between 15 and 22 percent of their budget setting up the administrative system demanded by managed care organizations and other insurers. For example, as competition for managed care contracts intensifies, hospitals are expanding their administrative staffs about eight times faster than their nursing staffs (Hilzenrath 1994a). Hospital advertising is also up over 11 percent (Gordon 1995). Physicians are experiencing similar increases in their administrative costs as well (Hilzenrath 1994b.)

The expansion of Medicare managed care is also pushing up administrative costs. Medicare's administrative costs are much lower than those of private insurers (Iglehart 1992). Consequently, as the elderly switch from Medicare to private managed care, overall administrative costs rise.

Profits in the health care industry are soaring as well. For instance, profits in the drug industry are five times higher than the average profits of the Fortune 500 companies (Levy 1995). HMOs are also doing quite well (Ehart 1995a). They are not only piling up billions in cash, but their stock last year rose 32.7 percent, while the Standard and Poor's index of five hundred companies fell 1.5 percent. They also had a strong first quarter in 1995. (Freudenheim 1995c). Overall, health stock rose by about 10 percent last year. Further consolidations will likely result in even higher profits and stock prices.

Rising profits and other administrative expenses show up as health care expenditures on the ledgers of corporations and government agencies providing medical insurance, and they are included in the premiums of individual purchases. These expenses leave less for clinical services. One economist observed, "What is supposed to be a movement toward greater efficiency and a streamlining of costs . . . may actually turn out to be a boondoggle for administration" (Hilzenrath 1994a). The counterargument is that the gains in clinical efficiency outweigh the costs of extra administration and profits. This counterargument suggests that there is some conflict between the trends in our system today. Recall that we had in fact scored managed care positively for reducing the overutilization of services. Here we must score the expansion of managed care in both private and public sectors negatively for its effects on administrative costs. We give a score of −2.0 for this criterion. We note incidentally that the market-based Michel bill received a positive score in chapter 4 on this criterion, recognizing some specific measures it would have required to lower administrative costs.

Tough Contractual Bargaining

Trends in our current system are increasing the use of tough bargaining with doctors and hospitals, especially as managed care organizations (MCOs) become larger buyers of services (Anders and Winslow 1995). For example, by limiting the size of their networks, managed care organizations gain a larger percentage of their doctors' practices and greater control over their fees (Ehart 1995b). As consolidations reduce the competition among MCOs, doctors are being squeezed even harder (Pearsall 1995). Many are in fact selling their private practice to insurance companies and large managed care corporations (Whitlow 1995). Some hospitals find themselves in similar situations (Peterson 1994). As we noted in discussion of the previous criterion, a significant portion of the savings derived from this tough bargaining goes into marketing, management, and profit.

Employers in turn are getting firm with managed care organizations that have tried to keep the savings from discounts for themselves (Battagliola 1994). For example, in an effort to lower HMO prices, ten large businesses, led by American Express and Merrill Lynch, recently combined their purchases of employee health care coverage. This joint purchase of $1 billion in twenty-seven markets should greatly enhance their bargaining power. Ten more large employers may soon join the group (Freudenheim 1995d). Small businesses are also discovering "the power of pooling" and forming voluntary purchasing groups (Maynard 1995). In San Francisco, Minnesota, Houston, Cleveland, and other selected cities, employers are setting up purchasing cooperatives. But how tough they actually get is another matter. During the 1980s, business health coalitions claimed all sorts of savings through tough bargaining that did not materialize, because it is very difficult for ten or twenty corporations, with different policies and boards, to work in unison.

This type of tough bargaining with managed care organizations is also occurring in the public sector. To cite one case, the California Public Employees Retirement System (CALPERS), which represents 900,000 workers and their dependents, recently negotiated a 2.5 to 4.0 percent price reduction from some of the state's largest HMOs. This came after CALPERS publicly criticized the HMOs for spending about 20 percent of their revenues on profits, marketing, and administrative expenses, including multimillion dollar executive salaries (Anders 1995a). Yet, such examples are few and cover a small fraction of public employees. Instead, most public sector bargaining is aimed at employees, attempting to increase their out-of-pocket contributions.

In response to tough bargaining by managed care organizations, some practitioners have formed their own managed care groups ("Physician Corp. of America to Buy Health Plus" 1994). For example, New Jersey recently licensed its first two physician-owned HMOs with networks that include thousands of doctors from across the state. Other doctors are countering the power of managed care organizations by joining unions. According to the American Medical Association (AMA), three-quarters of the nation's private practitioners have signed managed care contracts, and nearly all individually negotiated them. To help, a group of private practitioners have formed a union. Similar unions in other states are also trying to increase the clout of their members. In the words of the president of one such union in California, "the days of the Lone Ranger have ended" (Valdez-Dapena 1995, p. 101). Hospitals are also banding together to increase their influence as well (Jacobs 1995).

The AMA has also initiated a national campaign for any willing provider (AWP) legislation (Offner 1994). The AMA is pushing states, as well as the federal government, to enact laws forcing MCOs to accept into their network any licensed health care provider who agrees to abide by its rules and payment schedules. By greatly expanding their networks and denying them the ability to exclude specific providers, AWP legislation would significantly reduce the power of MCOs.

According to most indications, bargaining between buyers and sellers in the health care marketplace has become more stringent. Consequently, this criterion receives a score of +3.0. We do note three potential trouble spots. First, only large buyers are engaging in tough bargaining with their sellers, and many of these sellers are themselves getting bigger. In other words, tough bargaining has not reached a large portion of the population or providers. Second, this tough bargaining has not resulted in overall price reductions. A decline in the general inflation rate, not tough bargaining between buyers and sellers, is primarily responsible for falling health care prices (Light 1994e). If physicians organize to counter bargaining in larger blocks, tough bargaining may cause price increases.

Minimizing Cost Shifting

Out-of-pocket expenditures continue to increase and shift costs to workers, retirees, and their families. Declining health benefits is another form of cost shifting (Nixon 1994). Cutbacks in Medicare and Medicaid have similar effects (Findlay 1995). For example, the elderly now pay 50 percent more of their income on health care than they did before Medicare started (Merline 1995). Also, as the elderly choose low-cost, low-coverage managed care plans, some health care costs, which were previously paid by Medicare, now are paid by them (Toner and Pear 1995). On the supply side, low Medicare reimbursements force providers to move costs to other patients. And tough bargaining by large purchasers compels providers to charge more to other, less powerful customers. For example, CALPERS or Stanford University's gains are shifted to smaller employers in the Bay Area.

Despite all the rhetoric, health care costs are still rising over twice as fast as the general inflation rate (Light 1994e). Moreover, large buyers with substantial monopsony power appear to be putting these costs on weaker buyers or payers. The dynamics of the market may look like this: Large corporations decrease their costs through managed care. Large managed care organizations decrease their costs through discounted provider payments. Providers charge other insurance plans, such as smaller managed care networks or indemnity plans, higher fees to help offset the discount. These insurers then charge their customers higher premiums. Smaller businesses, facing these higher premiums, increase the costs to their employees. The "success" of managed competition may be more like squeezing the balloon of health care spending, so that while costs go down for large buyers, the costs to everyone else expand.

Managed care has its own unique forms of cost shifting. For example, health care providers, such as hospitals and physicians, forced to discount prices for managed care organizations, charge indemnity plans more (Quint 1995). As managed care grows and the fee-for-service sector shrinks, such cost shifting will become more difficult but still quite prevalent in hidden differences between one managed care contract and another. Of course, "cherry picking" of enrollees in managed care is also another form of cost shifting from the healthy to the sick. A major form of apparent savings through cost shifting is taking place in Medicare managed care contracts. Corporations are focusing on areas where the Medicare rates are high. Since they get 95 percent of these rates (rather than competitive bidding), they are making 20 to 30 percent profit on gross revenues, an almost unheard of amount that has led some to call Medicare contracts the largest "welfare program" in government for investors. This selective marketing leaves Medicare paying for unmanaged costs in all other markets. Further, managed care companies can to some degree sign up healthier customers, thus shifting still more costs back to Medicare (Merline 1995).

The most obvious, and perhaps the most disturbing, form of cost shifting is the increasing number of uninsured and the "dumping" of these patients onto the public sector where providers and public hospitals cannot impose their costs on anyone else (Mann et al. 1994). Consequently, the uninsured are receiving less free care (Weiner 1994).

For all these reasons, this criterion receives a score of -2.0.

Anti–Fraud and Abuse

There are some indications that both fraud and abuse are flourishing in the highly competitive and volatile medical market. For example, most states are currently enrolling their Medicaid populations into mandatory managed care. However, in some of these states, aggressive marketers, who work on commission, are using fraudulent tactics, such as bribery, forgery, and misrepresentation, to enroll people into their HMOs (Sugg 1995). In fact, marketing and other kinds of abuse are increasing throughout the managed care industry (Olmos 1995). Some types of insurance fraud appear to be on the rise (Yarborough 1995). Meanwhile, efforts to reduce provider fraud have greatly increased. What seems to get little attention are the analogous forms of underpayment or underservice by insurers, although both are probably rising (Light 1994a).

In light of these growths, anti–fraud and abuse measures remain largely inadequate. Some states, like Maryland, have launched investigations (Sugg 1995), and the Justice Department recently formed a task force to study the problem (Olmos 1995). But these efforts represent no significant change from last year.

The score on this criterion is -0.5 to register our concern about the modest evidence of increasing fraud and abuse.

The average score for benchmark 7 is -0.4. Given the quite divergent scores for individual criteria, it is more important to look at the individual criteria than the average.

Benchmark 8: Public Accountability

We evaluate this benchmark on the basis of four criteria: (1) availability of explicit, public, and detailed procedures for assessing plans and practitioners; (2) explicit and democratic procedures for allocation decisions; (3) fair grievance procedures; and (4) protection of privacy.

Explicit Public Procedures for Evaluation

In an increasingly anti-government climate, public oversight and regulatory requirements are largely inadequate and declining. For example, in most states there is little regulation of HMOs after their initial certification (Pearsall 1995). At the same time, greater consolidation and the birth of huge conglomerates—large, vertically integrated health care systems—are privatizing evaluation and accountability. These for-profit health care delivery systems are accountable only to their stockholders. Consequently, when local community hospitals, which are directly accountable to the public, close or merge with the for-profits, public accountability declines. Also, if part of the federal government, such as the Federal Drug Administration, turns some of its responsibilities over to the private sector, public accountability is further reduced (Burros 1995).

There are some private sector efforts to increase accountability, however. For example, the HMO industry and its National Committee for Quality Assurance are publishing "report cards," which evaluate health insurance plans using standardized measures for quality and cost (Winslow 1995b). These report cards could eventually raise the standards of care throughout the industry (Quinn 1994). Moreover, these private accountability and quality systems are moving toward specific outcome measures.

Nevertheless, these evaluations are largely based on self-grading, and their evaluation procedures are not publicly disclosed. The public is only informed of the results. Their databases, which the industry claims contain trade secrets, are considered private property, so that some of the best information about the health of the nation is publicly inaccessible (Winslow 1994).

Even some public measures aimed at improving public accountability are not open to the public. For example, the National Practitioner Data Bank, which was established by Congress to collect data on malpractice and disciplinary actions, recently issued its first report. Although hospitals must consult the data bank before granting doctors staff privileges, the public has no access to it.

In our discussion of this criterion in chapter 5, we noted the important steps toward evaluation and public accountability that were taken by some of the plans. This modest effort of the private sector falls short of the kind of accountability needed, and the rapid expansion of managed care since our baseline year makes the problem all the more urgent. We score this criterion a −2.0.

Explicit Democratic Procedures for Resource Allocation

The trends toward expansion of managed care and increased corporatization of health care delivery means more and more allocation decisions affecting large numbers of people will be made by managers with no accountability to and no imput from the public. Only fears of tort litigation act as a public constraint on resource allocation decisions.

Some leading HMOs are undertaking more careful institutional evaluations of new technologies in making decisions about coverage for them. This process is, however, viewed entirely as a proprietary decision. In some cases, corporations that conduct safety and efficacy assessments of new technologies sell their results to managed care organizations and other insurers. But all of these transactions involve no explicit democratic procedures. Given the rapid rate of technology dissemination and the pressures to contain costs, decisions of this sort are being made more frequently, and relatively more power and discretion are accumulating in the hands of corporations and managers as compared to practitioners and their patients.

There has never been a system of fair democratic procedures for re-source allocation decisions in the private sector and only rare experiments in that direction in the public sector (e.g., Oregon; see Daniels 1991). The fact that nothing is emerging as a result of current trends might suggest we simply score this criterion a zero. Nevertheless, we score the trends a −1.0 to indicate our concern that locus of decision making is shifting more than ever to managed care providers and other insurers and away from any context in which patient input, let alone public input and accountability, is recognized as important.

Fair Grievance Procedures

There is little evidence that managed care organizations have voluntarily instituted adequate grievance procedures, and certainly no measurable moves in that direction since our baseline year (Stayn 1994). Managed care organizations generally do not install an ombudsman, and most retain the ability to dismiss physicians "without cause" and without an adequate ap-peals process. Extralegal forms of dispute resolution of the sort provided by fair grievance procedures are an important way of reducing reliance on tort litigation. There is proof that more health-related disputes are being settled using a variety of alternative dispute resolution techniques and, according to *The Wall Street Journal*, results are generally superior to those obtained through the traditional court system (Felsenthal 1994). In the case of disagreements about the use of medical services that are urgently needed or desired by someone, an alternative to tort litigation is clearly desirable. The reluctance of rapidly expanding and increasingly corporatized man-aged care organizations to voluntarily institute grievance procedures contin-ues to force a reliance on the courts.

As in the scoring of the previous criterion, we show our concern about the rapidly growing need for these procedures by assigning a −1.0 to this criterion, even though the health care system has always lacked adequate grievance procedures.

Adequate Privacy Protection

The rapid development of managed care, as well as advances in com-puter technology, means that massive amounts of personal information are now available online, and this trend is accelerating. While restricting access to these electronic medical records may actually be easier than limiting access to their more traditional counterparts, privacy protections still remain inadequate (R. Davis 1995). For example, few federal laws specifically restrict the unauthorized use of this information. However, the Federal Trade Commission, in an agreement with the Medical Information Bureau, recently gave 15 million Americans greater access to their electronic medical records (Birnbaum 1995). But without adequate safeguards, these growing databases threaten everyone's privacy. As part of managed care, medical reviewers want to know more and more about patients' conditions, prognosis, and treatments. Patients are legitimately concerned about their privacy, especially in the area of mental health (Henderson 1994).

Because of this predicament, and the absence of adequate measures to address it, this criterion receives a score of −1.0. We note that the market-based Michel bill received a low but positive score of 1.0 for this criterion because it gave modest recognition to the problem.

The average score for this benchmark is −1.25.

Benchmark 9: Comparability

This benchmark requires that an overall health budget be constructed on either the national or state level, so that it can be compared with other spending priorities. In other words, this benchmark calls for the establishment of an accounting of health care spending that facilitates trade-offs between health care and other needed goods and services. The major trends in our system do not change it from what we had in the baseline year, namely, no adequate mechanism to establish comparability. We score this benchmark a zero.

Benchmark 10: Degree of Consumer Choice

Criteria for this benchmark concern the degree to which people can make fully informed choices of their primary-care providers, their specialists, other licensed providers, and specific health care procedures.

Choice of Primary-Care Provider

The growth of managed care is affecting different people differently. For example, Medicaid receipts, who usually have difficulty finding doctors willing to treat them, generally experience greater choice under managed care. With mandatory enrollment in Medicaid managed care on the rise, the number of people who fall into this category is steadily growing. Previously uninsured people who are now insured also have greater choice of primary-care providers. But the dominant trend is clearly in the other direction—more uninsured and less care for the poor (Somerville

1994). People who are forced to move from fee-for-service care with indemnity insurance into managed care have significantly less choice— and this is the major category of people given current trends. People who can afford to retain fee-for-service care do so and retain better choice of all providers (Davis et al. 1995). Under managed care, where 30 percent of the providers treat 70 percent of the patients and strong financial incentives keep people "in network," choices are much more limited (Gorski 1995).

Restricted physician choice is also the leading reason most elderly are not joining Medicare HMOs (Schwartz 1995). The elderly highly value their relationship with their doctors, and many are reluctant to leave the fee-for-service arrangements of Medicare. On the other hand, some Republicans are pushing Medicare HMOs by arguing that they actually increase the choices of the elderly (Toner and Pear 1995). However, greater choice among insurance plans is not the same as greater choice of physician (Stovall, Hughes, and Schwartz 1994). It is the latter that the elderly clearly seem to prefer.

Within managed care, choice of primary-care and other providers is affected by the frequent dismissal and replacement of providers. Insurance companies and managed care organizations can drop doctors from their network with little or no explanation or warning. This "deselection," as the industry calls it, not only disrupts care but forces some enrollees to choose another primary-care provider. While there are few national statistics on turnover rates in HMO networks, the practice is causing some apprehension (Neus 1995).

Choice of primary-care provider is also affected by employer choices of health care plans and decisions to change them. When employers seek another plan for their own goals, usually to lower costs, sick employees may have to terminate treatment with a given provider or clinic, and many employees will have to switch primary-care providers if the new plan does not include their original provider. The problem is particularly acute because most employers offer their employees only one plan (Employee Benefit Research Institute 1994), thus restricting choice even when no switches are made.

To score this criterion, we must weigh different trends against each other. On the whole, the growth of managed care and the increased reliance of employers on it seem to reduce choice of primary-care providers. The rising number of uninsured also means more people have no choice of primary-care providers. We therefore score this criterion a −1.0. Note that there is less choice according to this criterion, yet the system as a whole is relying more on primary care, a fact reflected when we scored the criterion in benchmark 6 concerning primary care a +2.0. We also note for comparison that the market-based Michel bill received a +0.5 on this criterion for benchmark 10 in chapter 5 because it increased choice for some poor people by proposing increased access to community and migrant health centers.

Choice of Specialists

The same considerations that apply to choice of primary-care providers also apply to the choice of specialists, but because managed care organizations specifically aim to *reduce* access to specialty care (while increasing it to primary care), the problem is worse. For this reason, we score this criterion a −1.5.

Choice of Other Health Care Providers

Managed care significantly limits patients' choices of such mainstream providers as hospitals and physical therapists. Managed care organizations decide which hospitals their enrollees can use, when they can use them, and for how long. The same is true for physical therapists and other types of medical subspecialists.

Americans have always followed a pluralistic approach to health and have strongly supported an individual's right to choose among competing forms of health care (Lisa 1994). Today, over one-third of Americans (more than 60 million people) use at least one unconventional therapy. The most popular are chiropractic, relaxation techniques, and massage. Of the three, chiropractic is the largest, with over 45,000 practitioners and 20 million patients (Eisenberg et al. 1993). The ability of people to choose these kinds of providers is significantly limited by the expansion of managed care.

These limitations are largely financial. In some cases, previously covered services are either no longer covered or covered inadequately. The best example is chiropractic, which is covered under most fee-for-service plans, including Medicare and Medicaid (Caplan 1991). However, most managed care organizations either omit chiropractors from their provider network or allow them in a limited way (Caplan and Scarpaci 1989). Consequently, most enrollees seeking chiropractic care must pay for it themselves. As more chiropractic patients move from fee-for-service to managed care, many of them are forced to discontinue their care (Caplan 1993). Increasing out-of-pocket expenditures for mainstream medicine, which leaves less money for other uses, is having a similar effect on other alternative health care providers. These kinds of changes reduce peoples' ability to use alternative health care, even if it is their preferred choice of care. It is a bit ironic that these limitations are growing at a time when alternative health care is gaining legitimacy and enjoying many well-publicized successes (McKenna 1995).

Since we see the restrictions on choice of other providers as even more significant than the increasing restrictions on specialists, we score this criterion −2.0.

Choice of Procedure

Managed care providers rely on extremely detailed protocols or practice guidelines to limit the use of many services. There is even a market for commercial formulations of such guidelines. In many cases, these involve restrictions on procedures that physicians and their patients would have preferred.

Some of these restrictions are clearly legitimate attempts to limit the use of ineffective or experimental techniques. Some try to curtail over-

Table 6-1   Benchmarks of Fairness for Current Trends in United States Health Care

Benchmark 1:	
Universal Coverage and Participation	
Mandatory Coverage and Participation	−1.0
Portability	−0.5
Average Score for Benchmark 1	−0.75*
Benchmark 2:	
Minimizing Nonfinancial Barriers	
Minimizing Maldistributions	−1.0
Reform of Health Professional Education	2.0
Minimizing Language, Culture, Class Barriers	0.0
Minimizing Educational and Informational Barriers	0.0
Average Score for Benchmark 2	0.25
Benchmark 3:	
Comprehensive and Uniform Benefits	
Comprehensiveness	No Score
Reduced Tiering and Uniform Quality	1.0
Average Score for Benchmark 3	1.0*
Benchmark 4:	
Equitable Financing—Community-Rated Contributions	
True Community-rated Premiums	−0.5
Minimum Discrimination via Cash Payments	0.0
Average Score for Benchmark 4	−0.25
Benchmark 5:	
Equitable Financing—By Ability to Pay	0.0
Benchmark 6:	
Value For Money—Clinical Efficacy	
Emphasis on Primary Care	2.0
Emphasis on Public Health and Prevention	−1.0
Systematic Assessment of Outcomes	0.5

utilization. Their effect, however, is to reduce the choice of procedures available. It is reasonable to reply that some of these choices should be narrowed and that some limitations on choice do not in any way interfere with adequate treatment that reflects reasonable priorities in delivering health services to a whole population. This is true. Some patients are not entitled to some choices they currently make, and a system that limits these choices is not in itself less fair for doing so.

We find it difficult to believe, however, that all the kinds of restrictions now being imposed on the choice of procedures fall into this category. We doubt, in other words, that they all reflect defensible claims that only ineffective or cost-ineffective treatments are involved. We are particularly concerned because these limitations are the result of decisions made in

Table 6-1   (Continued)

Minimizing Overutilization and Underutilization	2.0
Average Score for Benchmark 6	0.9
Benchmark 7:	
Value For Money—Financial Efficacy	
Minimizing Administrative Overhead	−2.0
Tough Contractual Bargaining	3.0
Minimizing Cost Shifting	−2.0
Anti–Fraud and Abuse Measures	−0.5
Average Score for Benchmark 7	−0.4
Benchmark 8:	
Public Accountability	
Explicit Public Procedures for Evaluation	−2.0
Explicit Democratic Procedures for Resource Allocation	−1.0
Fair Grievance Procedures	−1.0
Adequate Privacy Protection	−1.0
Average Score for Benchmark 8	−1.25
Benchmark 9:	
Comparability	0.0
Benchmark 10:	
Degree of Consumer Choice	
Choice of Primary-Care Provider	−1.0
Choice of Specialists	−1.5
Choice of Other Health Care Providers	−2.0
Choice of Procedure	−2.5
Average Score for Benchmark 10	−1.75
TOTAL: Average across Fully Scored Benchmarks	−0.3

Explanation of scores: Current health care trends were judged according to how much they are increasing or decreasing the fairness of the U.S. health care system. A score of zero represents no change from the baseline, the summer of 1994. Scores range from −5.0 to +5.0. An asterisk indicates incomplete scoring.

ways that are not publicly accountable (as noted in benchmark 8). This leaves us with the conclusion that choice of procedures is being significantly reduced, and some important but hard to estimate portion of that reduction is for choices people should be making for themselves. Given the rapid expansion of the organizations restricting these choices and the range of choices affected, we score this criterion a −2.5. This provisional scoring might be revised upward if explicit, adequate reasons for the limitations were given.

The average score for benchmark 10 is −1.75.

Conclusion

All ten benchmarks are summarized in table 6–1.

We had two goals in this chapter. One goal was to illustrate a use of the benchmarks different from the one in chapters 4 and 5. There we asked how reform proposals would alter the system relative to the status quo. In this chapter, we have asked how current trends at work in the system affect fairness on the ten dimensions of our matrix. We had to modify the scale and slightly alter the criteria used in scoring the benchmarks. We hope that the attempt to apply the criteria to these trends would force us and the reader to bring assumptions out in the open that bear on judgments about fairness and to identify information we still need to be more confident about the judgments we make. We expect the application is provocative and will stimulate debate, criticism, reconsideration of assumptions, and the gathering of additional information. If it has these effects, then we have demonstrated the value of the tool we are trying to develop.

A second goal in this chapter was to show the urgency of considering the effects of current trends on the fairness of an already quite unfair system. Some changes have a positive effect on fairness, but many do not. Indeed, the average score for eight of ten benchmarks of the current trends is −0.3. If we disguise this fact by referring to all the changes as "reforms," then we hide from ourselves some of their real effects. The extent and significance of these changes goes beyond their immediate effect on fairness, as measured by our benchmarks. Indeed, they force us to face a question we have not yet raised: Do the changes now taking place make it harder to secure fairness in our system? Do they make it more difficult to undertake reforms that would make the system more fair? We turn to these questions briefly in the final chapter.

7

Prospects for Fair Reform

Applying the benchmarks of fairness to current changes in our health care system, as we did in chapter 6, yields the provisional judgment that our system is becoming less fair in important ways. This judgment is provisional because the evidence about these trends is incomplete and because the time period during which the trends were assessed is so short. A larger question is raised, however, by the scope and speed of the trends we surveyed, especially the rapid expansion of managed care and the corporatization of larger sectors of our health care system. These trends fundamentally alter the organization of our delivery system. Perhaps more important, they change in basic ways the culture that has pervaded our delivery system throughout this century. Will these trends and the changes they produce in the attitudes and values of those who organize and deliver health care make the system harder to reform fairly in the long run? Will reform that would score highly on our ten benchmarks be more difficult to achieve?

To focus these questions more clearly, let us imagine that the current trends operating in our system continue over the next decade or so. Specifically, we are imagining the following. Government cost-cutting measures restrict the growth of Medicare and Medicaid budgets and force significant numbers of the elderly and most Medicaid recipients into managed care arrangements. At the same time, cost-containing measures by employers and aggressive expansion of for-profit managed care organizations push the majority of Americans into one form or another of managed care. Only a fairly wealthy group of insurance buyers can afford indemnity coverage for fee-for-service coverage. Because strong antigovernment sentiment continues, partly because the middle class feels particularly squeezed out of any share in the country's economic growth, there is no expansion of public insurance programs for the rising number of uninsured. This is caused by some employers continuing to reduce benefits and the world of full-time jobs is being replaced by "a temporary or sub-contracting nether world . . . a just-in-time, bare-bones and cheaper work force . . . seeping like a mist into every corner of American livelihood" (Ansberry 1993). The provision of medical care to the uninsured becomes more difficult for two reasons. Public hospitals and clinics are forced to close (Sack 1995) as a result of public budget cuts and continued resistance to tax increases. Moreover, shifting the costs of unreimbursed services to other buyers of health care services becomes harder in a more competitive, managed care world.

Our point in imagining this scenario is not to make a stronger extrapolation of our judgments about the fairness of current trends than we were able to make in chapter 6. Rather, we want to see if the changes wrought by these trends make the system more or less amenable to efforts aimed at fair reform. We believe that there are ways to flesh out the details of this scenario that support both optimistic and pessimistic conclusions about the possibilities of fair reform. Our point in this exercise is not to pretend that we are professional seers, however, but to show that, whatever happens, the need to assess the available options for reform in light of our benchmarks will remain.

Let us begin with the bad news first, the more pessimistic interpretation of our scenario. One feature of the scenario is the vast concentration of economic power in the hands of for-profit, managed care corporations. We can imagine that there will be considerable shake-out of local health care providers. The kinds of capital needed for the formation of significant networks of providers will produce many large-scale mergers of the sort we have increasingly seen since the failure of reform in the 103rd Congress. Thousands of local, small-scale physicians' groups, clinics, and hospitals will be bought out and amalgamated into large, investor-driven corporations.

This concentration of power has implications for the possibility of some reforms. If most of the health care system is consolidated into a few managed care organizations that structure services for a given area, any reform proposals ignoring or threatening them will have to fight the full opposition of this industry. This kind of opposition from entrenched interests is formidable and has already shaped the health care debate. To cite one case, Clinton thought it politically infeasible to support any form of single-payer system, such as the McDermott/Wellstone proposal, since the insurance industry would have blocked it using their wealth and power. With consolidation of power in the hands of those who control managed care, an even larger force is arrayed against certain types of reform. Many previously independent health care providers and physicians, who had sometimes opposed the interests of insurers and favored the interests of patients, will be unable to act as a counterpoint to the managed care industry. Consequently, proposals that scored highly on our benchmarks, like the single-payer or the heavily managed competition proposals, may seem politically unattractive. The pessimistic interpretation of the scenario suggests that comprehensive reform of that sort has forever been moved beyond the pale in our system.

The strength of this pessimistic interpretation can be brought out if we think in more detail about the effects of managed care on physicians and other clinical providers. Many physicians and other clinical providers will have become increasingly enmeshed economically in the fortunes of managed care organizations. Many clinical practices would be bought by managed care networks. These clinicians will work for the industry under attack by some reforms; they will be paid to advance the economic interests of that industry. A whole generation of practitioners will have become acclimated to the culture and socialized into the ethos of managed care organizations. For example, some of the support expressed by associations of primary-care and other physicians for a Canadian-style single-payer system, in which their autonomy would have been preserved, will be undermined if the dominant experience of physicians in our society is that of managed care. If they come to identify with the interests of the managed care organizations for which they work, then they may see "government regulation" as a threat to them rather than as a protection for patients.

Of course, there is an alternative gloss on this aspect of the scenario, a version of "the worse, the better." Some may believe that physicians will soon grow to resist the loss of clinical autonomy in many managed care systems and will eagerly welcome the prospect of a government-run system like Canada's, or that they will welcome a more "patient-focused" set of regulatory reforms. They will have learned, so the argument goes, what is really good for them.

We believe, however, that this crystallization of practitioner support for a single-payer system, or for a more government-regulated form of managed care, will not be the dominant result of the hegemony of managed care. Instead, we think that incentives will work to increase physician support for managed care culture. We also think that in the better parts of the managed care system, and there will be some excellent examples of managed care, there need be no deep conflict between a patient-centered ethic by physicians and the goals of a well run managed care system. The unpredictable element is the balance that will be achieved between well run and badly run managed care systems.

Even if this pessimistic interpretation of the scenario reduces the prospects of the highest-scoring forms of reform, such as the single-payer plan, it leaves the door open to many other elements of reform that were on the agenda in the 103rd Congress. Powerful managed care systems may compromise quality of care for higher profits. The public may become suspicious of them because of their lack of accountability (Daniels and Sabin 1995). We already know, even before our imagined scenario has fully developed, that all is not perfect with the managed care experience. According to surveys, the millions of Americans who fiercely clung to "choice" and feared government-run health care appear at present to be satisfied with the managed care they receive, whether they have been forced into it by employers, by the cost of alternatives, or by public insurance programs. If one looks more closely, however, they are happier about lower out-of-pocket costs and somewhat less satisfied with less choice and longer waits. If one looks still closer, at the minority of enrollees who are sick enough to be treated by specialists, the picture looks even worse. A national survey found that compared to those in traditional unmanaged care, sick patients in managed care were 3.3 times more likely to report that they received inappropriate care, 4.0 times more likely to report that their examination was not thorough, 2.5 times more likely to report they had inadequate time with their physician, and 2.1 times more likely to report that the doctor did not care (RWJ 1995). Although these are patient perceptions and do not necessarily mean that their medical care was inferior, doctors and nurses in mature managed care markets, where utilization rates were already low by 1990, are reporting staff reductions and deskilling that they believe cause mistakes and deaths.

Even if we have to take the power of managed care as a given, there may be considerable room for improvement of its worst features. Such reforms would involve government regulation, reducing the use of waiting periods, exclusion clauses, and biased selection (benchmark 4); providing subsidies for the uninsured to buy coverage (benchmark 5); forcing more accountability of performance and decision making (benchmark 8); requiring adequacy in benefit packages (benchmark 3); and providing for across-plan assessment of outcomes and quality measurement (benchmark 6). The power of managed care may thus significantly limit our options, but it leaves considerable room for improvement elsewhere.

There is, however, a somewhat more optimistic interpretation of our general scenario. The organizational changes the scenario involves may also produce cultural changes that enhance the possibility of further, and fairer, reforms. For example, one important source of opposition to comprehensive reform in the past—and this includes the 1940s, the 1970s, and the 103rd Congress—has been the fear of many Americans, encouraged by opponents of any reform (Center for Public Integrity 1994; Kolbert 1995; Carlson and McLeod 1994; Reinhardt 1995a), that they would lose choice and quality of care if "big government" ran or regulated the health care system. But the scenario we imagine means that most Americans *will already have experienced the changes they most feared*. Moreover, some change is quite positive. In our scenario, the system will squeeze out a lot of overpricing and waste; it will improve the pay and increase the supply of primary-care doctors quickly; it will encourage employers to ignore their differences and form buying cooperatives; it will lead to more attention to effectiveness and even cost effectiveness in clinical interventions. These changes are painful for many and to the extent that they are behind us, they no longer form a basis for opposition to reforms that in the past would have hastened them.

To the extent that many Americans find their health care system satisfactory, because it is performing reasonably well, they may have less opposition to modest regulatory reforms that eliminate the rougher edges. To the extent that they find the system seriously compromising quality, coverage for needed benefits, and choice of procedures and doctors, the source of their unhappiness will not be the government, as they had feared, but the relatively unregulated medical market and the powerful medical insurers and managed care organizations. The public may then be more amenable to a bigger regulatory role of government in assuring quality, accountability, and adequate benefits. Ironically, some system of reforms resembling those embedded in the Clinton plan, which scored reasonably well on many benchmarks, might seem more politically palatable down the road than it did in 1994.

To make this optimistic suggestion more plausible, it is worth describing in more detail how the general scenario may affect the experience of Americans. Nearly all Americans, both providers and patients, will have been incorporated into organized delivery systems that operate on fixed budgets. Being in such delivery systems gradually works to alter a deep-seated culture of autonomy and choice, including the demand for "the best care at any cost," replacing it with one of management and value for money. This cultural change sets the stage for accepting *reasonable* limits on the availability of services. One of the biggest fears the American public expressed in thinking about government-run reform, including "premium caps" or global budgets, was the fear of limits or rationing. Within the Clinton Health Care Task Force, the Ethics Working Group had the White House undertake a more explicit discussion of rationing and the ethical issues it involves. The Ethics Group was told that cost saving would make rationing unnecessary and that the "R word" should be avoided in all memos and documents for fear that it would be used to attack the plan.

The introduction of limits is given legitimacy in our scenario because it is being done by the right people, the private sector, rather than the wrong people, the government. No other country that has succeeded in holding down its health care costs while providing prompt, excellent services to all residents has subjected patients and doctors to so much regulation as do managed care corporations. Corporate-sponsored health care reform—dare we call it "corporate socialism"?—is turning out to be much more extreme, but also much more acceptable, because government is not doing it.

Still, the limits are not so tolerable to sick patients who know they need services that are denied them. As long as patients think that profits and not patient welfare motivate corporate decisions about care, then limits will be challenged by patients and providers, either by "gaming" the system or by resorting to tort litigation. In earlier chapters, we talked about the importance of fair, publicly accountable decision making about resources, better grievance procedures, and greater accountability concerning the performance of managed care organizations. These elements of benchmark 8 and, to some extent, of benchmarks 3 and 6 are all made more reasonable targets of regulatory reform once people more widely experience the shortcomings of a system that lacks such protections.

Consider another example of the greater legitimacy that private change seems to have brought with it compared to government-imposed change. A government-sponsored effort to emphasize primary care and limit access to specialty care would have met strenuous political opposition from specialists. Patients would have feared that the government was keeping them from higher quality, necessary care. For example, when an effort to alter Medicare and Medicaid reimbursement rates in favor of primary-care doctors was made several years ago, surgeons and other specialists fought hard to retain their favored position. As a result, changes in reimbursements had to be tempered, even though that meant setting aside a sound economic rationale for more dramatically altered rates.

Managed care corporations, however, are creating a strong foundation of primary care, with a gatekeeper referral system for specialty care and hospitalization. These firms are changing the pay and market worth of primary-care doctors at the same time as oversupply is lowering the specialists' compensation. This corrects a major source of cost inflation, waste, unnecessary procedures, and poor coordination in the American health care system. Over time, it may lead to broader public acceptance, including physicians, of the central importance of primary care to health care organization and delivery. And, it may lead to greater acceptance of nonphysician clinicians to do the work for which board-certified physicians are overqualified. Cultural acceptance of these changes may even mean managed care organizations can take on the thicket of licensing laws that have long obstructed more cost effective use of personnel.

Still, many of these alterations can and probably will bring with them serious compromises in the quality of care. We commented in earlier chapters about the threat to quality that accompanies inappropriate deskilling of services. The changes can also involve a hidden thinning of the benefits available to people, a thinning of coverage not perceptible until we are sick and in need of services that are declared unnecessary or inappropriate by managed care protocols.

A public that becomes accustomed to limits but that resents unfair and unreasonable ones may consent to forms of government regulation that once seemed too intrusive. More specifically, they may come to support some elements of the reform proposals that were rejected by the 103rd Congress, particularly, those with relatively high benchmark scores. Because of broad experience with managed care and corporatization, the public may be less vulnerable to fear mongering and biased lobbying. People will be less likely to confuse the reform with the problem, that is, less inclined to confuse proposals to regulate managed care with the forces that led to their expansion. Or so the optimistic interpretation of our scenario suggests.

The fact that people are less likely to confuse the reform with the problem means, we believe, that the most important reform we could undertake, mandating universal insurance coverage, has a good chance of eventually being enacted. This is not a reform the market can do for us. Even if market reform produces some cost savings, or some reduction in the rate of increase of costs, which is still questionable in the long run, it cannot solve the problem of a growing uninsured population. Once people no longer blame efforts to achieve universal coverage for pushing them into managed care systems, it may become more possible to appeal to their sense of fairness.

We make no predictions about whether optimistic or pessimistic interpretations of our general scenario are more plausible. Either way, there is still a great need for fair reform of the system and careful assessment of the fairness of the options still open to us. That brings us back to our benchmarks and our point in developing them. The benchmarks help us connect our deepest social commitments about fairness to the complex details of health care reform. By injecting fairness into the debate about health care reform, and by helping think more rigorously about it, the tool we have shaped improves our prospects of achieving a fair health care system.

References

Aaron, H. J., and W. B. Schwartz. 1993. "Managed Competition: Little Cost Containment Without Budget Limits." *Health Affairs* 12(supp.):204–15.

Abraham, L. K. 1993. *Mama Might Be Better Off Dead*. Chicago: University of Chicago Press.

Aday, L. 1992. *At Risk in America: The Health and Health Care Needs of Vulnerable Populations in the United States*. New York: Basic Books.

Altman, D. E. 1995. "The Realities Behind the Polls." *Health Affairs* 14, no. 1:24–6.

Anders, George. 1995a. "CALPERS Gets Some HMOs to Cut Its Rates after Talks about Profit Margins Pay." *The Wall Street Journal*, February 9, p. B6.

———. 1995b. "Once a Hot Specialty, Anesthesiology Cools as Insurers Scale Back." *The Wall Street Journal*, March 17, pp. 1, A4.

Anders, George, and Hilary Stout. 1994. "Dose of Reform; with Congress Stalled, Health Care Is Shaped by the Private Sector." *The Wall Street Journal*, August 26, p. A1.

Anders, George, and Ron Winslow. 1995. "The HMO Trend: Big, Bigger, Biggest." *The Wall Street Journal*, March 30, pp. B1,4.

Ansberry, C. 1993. "Workers Are Forced to Take More Jobs with Few Benefits." *The Wall Street Journal*, March 11, A1, 9.

Arneson, R. 1988. "Equality and Equal Opportunity for Welfare." *Philosophical Studies* 54:79–95.

Baker, Steven R., and Stephen D. Brink. 1994. "Why We Need Quality Care Nationwide: Every Reform Plan Should Aim to Eliminate Inappropriate Care." *Business & Health*, April, p. 106.

Battagliola, Monica. 1994. "Pulling Together: By Buying in Groups, Employers Are Changing How Health Care is Delivered in Many Markets." *Business & Health*, April, p. 48.

Bayer, R. 1981. *Homosexuality and American Psychiatry: The Politics of Diagnosis*. Princeton N.J.: Princeton University Press.

Bell, Bertrand M. 1995. "Don't Just Privatize, But Rationalize New York City's Hospitals." *The New York Times*, March 7, pp. A12, 18.

Berk, M. L., and A. C. Mondheit. 1992. "The Concentration of Health Expenditures: An Update." *Health Affairs* 11, no. 4:145–9.

Binstock, Robert H. 1994. "Older Americans and Health Care Reform in the Nineties." in P. V. C. Rosenau, ed., *Health Care Reform in the Nineties*. Thousand Oaks, CA: Sage Publications, pp. 213–35.

Birnbaum, Jane. 1995. "Worried About Access to Insurance?" *The New York Times*, July 9, p. 9.

Blendon, R. J., M. Brodie, and J. Benson. 1995. "What Happened to Americans' Support for the Clinton Health Plan?" *Health Affairs* 14(summer):7–23.

Boren, S. D. 1994. "I Had a Tough Day Today, Hillary." *New England Journal of Medicine* 330:500–2.

Bradsher, Keith. 1995. "As 1 Million Leave Ranks of Insured, Debate Heats Up." *The New York Times*, August 27, pp. A1, 20.

Brand, N. 1992. "Learning to Use the Mediation Process—A Guide for Lawyers." *Arbitration Journal* 47:6–13.

Brock, D., and N. Daniels. 1994. "Ethical Foundations of the Clinton Administration's Proposed Health Care System." *JAMA* 271: 1189–1196.

Brown, Lawrence. 1994. "The Failure of Health Care Reform." Presentation of Community Health Program, Tufts University.

Buchanan, A., D. Brock, N. Daniels, and D. Wikler. 1996. *In the Shadow of Eugenics: The Human Genome Project and the Limits of Ethical Theory*. Unpublished manuscript.

Burner, S. T., D. R. Waldo, and D. R. McKusick. 1992. "National Health Expenditures: Projections through 2030." *Health Care Financing Review* 14:1–29.

Burros, Marian. 1995. "Congress Moving to Revamp Rules on Food Safety." *The New York Times*, July 3, pp. 1, 28.

Busack, Gary. 1994. "Rural Connections." *Health Progress* 75(April):48–50.

Calabresi, G., and P. Bobbitt. 1978. *Tragic Choices*. New York: W. W. Norton.

Califano, Joseph A. 1994. *Radical Surgery: What's Next for America's Health Care*. New York: Random House.

Callahan, D. 1987. *Setting Limits: Medical Goals in an Aging Society*. New York: Simon and Schuster.

Caplan, R. 1987. "The Clash over Quackery: Protecting Alternative Care." *Health/PAC Bulletin* 17(Winter):22–6.

———. 1988. "Holistic Health in the United States and the Changing Health Care Environment." *Holistic Medicine* 3:167–74.

———. 1991. "Health Care Reform and Chiropractic in the 1990's." *Journal of Manipulative and Physiological Therapeutics* 14(July/August):341–54.

———. 1993. "National Health Care Reform: At a Critical Crossroad" (Part One) *Journal of Chiropractic* 30(November):49–51.

Caplan, R., and J. Scarpaci. 1989. "The Consequences of Increased Competition on Alternative Health Care Practitioners in the United States." *Holistic Medicine* 4:125–35.

Carlson, E., and McLeod D. 1994. "The 'Big Lie' vs. Health Reform: Direct-Mail Firms 'Raised Millions' with Scare Letters." *AARP Newsletter* 35(1) Nov:9.

Carney, Leo. 1995. "Physicians Setting Up 2 HMOs." *The New York Times*, January 22, p. 1, 6.

Cohen, G. A. 1989. "On the Currency of Equality," *Ethics* 99:906–44.

Cohen, Joshua. 1995. "Amartya Sen: *Inequality Reexamined*." *Journal of Philosophy* 92, no. 5:275–288.

Coile, Russell C. 1990. *The New Medicine: Reshaping Medical Practice and Health Care Management*. Gaithersburg, Md.: Aspen Publishers.

Congressional Budget Office. 1992. *The Effects of Managed Care on the Use and Costs of Health Services*. Washington, D.C.: CBO.

———. 1993. *Managed Competition and Its Potential to Reduce Health Spending*. Washington, D.C.: CBO.

———. 1994. *An Analysis of the Managed Competition Act*. Washington, D.C.: CBO.

Conrad, P., and J. W. Schneider. 1992. *Deviance and Medicalization*. Philadelphia: Temple University Press.

"Consolidation Mania: Major Health Care Deals Surge to Record of $60 Billion." 1995. *Jenks Health Care Business Report* 5(January 24):1.

Cowley, Geoffrey, Susan Miller, and Mary Hager. 1995. "Intensive Care on a Budget." *Newsweek*, February 13, p. 86.

Crosson, Francis J. 1995. "Why Outcomes Measurement Must be the Basis for the Development of Clinical Guidelines." *Managed Care Quarterly* 3 (Spring):6–11.

Daniels, N. 1985. *Just Health Care*. Cambridge, England: Cambridge University Press.

———. 1988. *Am I My Parents' Keeper? An Essay on Justice between the Young and the Old*. New York: Oxford University Press.

———. 1990a. "Equality of What: Welfare, Resources, or Capabilities?" *Philosophy and Phenomenological Research* 50(supp.):273–96.

———. 1990b. "Insurability and the HIV Epidemic: Ethical Issues in Underwriting." *Milbank Quarterly* 68:497–526.

———. 1991. "Is the Oregon Rationing Plan Fair?" *JAMA* 265, 17:2232–35.

———. 1993. "Rationing Fairly: Programmatic Considerations." *Bioethics* 7, no. 2–3:224–33.

———. 1994. "The Articulation of Values and Principles Involved in Health Care Reform." *Journal of Medicine and Philosophy* 19:425–33.

———. 1995. *Seeking Fair Treatment: From the AIDS Epidemic to National Health Care Reform*. New York: Oxford University Press.

———. 1996. "Mental Disabilities, Equal Opportunity, and the ADA." In R. J. Bonnie, and J. Monahan, eds. *Mental Disorder, Work Disability, and the Law*. Chicago: University of Chicago Press (in press).

Daniels, N., and J. E. Sabin. 1991. "When Is Home Care Medically Necessary?" *Hastings Center Report* 21, no. 4:37–38.

———. 1995. "The Yin and Yang of Health Care System Reform." *Archives of Family Medicine* 4:67–71.

Daniels, N., D. Light, and R. Caplan. 1994. "Assessing The Fairness of National Health Care Reform" Princeton, NJ: Report to Robert Wood Johnson Foundation (Grant 20578).

Darling, Helen. 1995. "Market Reform: Large Corporations Lead the Way." *Health Affairs* 14(Spring):122–24.

Davis, Karen, Karen Scott Collins, Cathy Schoen, and Cynthia Morris. 1995. "Choice Matters: Enrollees' Views of Their Health Plans." *Health Affairs* 14(Summer):99–112.

Davis, M. 1995. "LA Fiscal Shock." *The Nation* 261(July 17/24):76.

Davis, Robert. 1995. "On Line 1995 Medical Records Raise Privacy Fears." *USA Today*, March 22, pp. 1–2.

De Lafuente, Della. 1994a. "Larger For-Profits Lead Solid in Rehab." *Modern Healthcare* 24(May 23):66.

———. 1994b. "Medical Groups Likely to Stay in Spotlight of Reform Efforts; Primary Care to Have Key Role." *Modern Healthcare* 24(January 3):42.

"Democrats, GOP Trade Charges over Medicare." 1995. *The Atlantic City Press*, July 29, p. A7.

Dubois, Robert, and Kevin Blank. 1995. "Bringing Clinical Accuracy to Provider Profiling Systems." *Managed Care Quarterly* 3:69–76.

Dworkin, R. 1994. "Will Clinton's Plan Be Fair?" *New York Review of Books* (January 13):20–25.

Eckholm, Eric, ed. 1993. *Solving America's Health Care Crisis*. New York: Random House.

———. 1994. "While Congress Remains Silent, Health Care Transforms Itself." *The New York Times*, December 18, p. 1, 34.

Ehart, William. 1995a. "Area HMOs Writing Prescriptions for Big Bucks." *The Press of Atlantic City*, March 26, p. 1, 5.

———. 1995b. "Side Effects of HMO 'Revolution' Often Felt By Doctors and Patients." *The Press of Atlantic City*, March 26, p. A5.

Eisenberg, D. M., R. C. Kessler, C. Foster, F. Horlock, D. Calkins, and T. Delbanco. 1993. "Unconventional Medicine in the United States—Prevalence, Costs, and Patterns of Use." *New England Journal of Medicine* 328:2466–52.

Employee Benefit Research Institute. 1995. "Sources of Health Insurance and Characteristics of the Uninsured." Special Report and Issue Brief #145, January. Washington, D.C.: Employee Benefit Research Institute.

Engelhardt, H. T. 1974. "Disease of Masturbation: Values and the Concept of Disease." *Bulletin of the History of Medicine* 48, no. 2:234–48.

———. 1986. *Foundations of Bioethics*. New York: Oxford University Press.

Enthoven, A. C. 1988. *Theory and Practice of Managed Competition in Health Care Finance*. Amsterdam: North-Holland.

———. 1993. "The History and Principles of Managed Competition." *Health Affairs* 12(supp.): 24–48.

Evans, R. G. 1993. "Health Care in the Canadian Community." In A. Bennett and O. Adams, eds. *Looking North for Health: What We Can Learn from Canada's Health Care System*. San Francisco, CA: Jossey-Bass, pp. 1–15.

Evans, R. G., M. L. Barer, and G. L. Stoddart. 1994. *Charging Peter to Pay Paul: Accounting for the Financial Effects of User Charges*. Ontario: The Premier's Council on Health, Well-being, and Social Justice.

Feingold, E. 1994. "Health Care Reform—More than Cost Containment and Universal Access." *American Journal of Public Health* 84:727–8.

Feldstein, P. J. 1994. *Health Policy Issues: An Economic Perspective on Health Care Reform*. Ann Arbor, MI: AUPHA Press/Health Administration Press.

Felsenthal, E. 1994. "What Happens When Patients Arbitrate Rather than Litigate?" *Wall Street Journal*, February 4, p. B1.

"Finding More Money for the Core of Public Health." 1994. *The Nation's Health* 24(January):1.

Findlay, Steven. 1995. "Entitlement Reform: The Time Has Come." *Business & Health* 13, January, p. 43.

Fisher, Ian, and Esther B. Fein. 1995. "Forced Marriage of Medicaid and Managed Care Hits Snags." *The New York Times*, August 28, p. B1, 5.

Fisher, Mary Jane. 1994. "Health Reform Bill Targets Problems Due to ERISA."

National Underwriter Life & Health—Financial Services Edition, February 20, p. 3.

Flood, A. B., D. P. Lorence, and J. Ding. 1993. "The Role of Expectations in Patients' Reports of Post-operative Outcomes and Improvement Following Therapy." *Medical Care* 31:1043–56.

Fowler, F. J. Jr., M. J. Barry, and G. Lu-Yau. 1993. "Patient Reported Complications and Follow-up Treatment after Radical Prostatectomy: The National Medicare Experience: 1988–1990 (Updated June 1993)." *Urology* 42(6):622–9.

Frank, Richard G. 1994. "Who Will Pay for Health Care Reform? Consequences of Redistribution of Funding for Mental Health Care." *JAMA* 272:1718.

Franks, P., C. M. Clancy, and M. R. Gold. 1993. "Health Insurance and Mortality: Evidence from a National Cohort." *JAMA* 270:737–41.

Freudenheim, Milt. 1995a. "Hospitals Are Tempted but Wary as For-Profits Chains Woo Them." *The New York Times*, January 4, p. A1.

———. 1995b. "States Shelving Ambitious Plans on Health Care." *The New York Times*, July 2, pp. A1, 20.

———. 1995c. "Penny-Pinching H.M.O.'s Showed Their Generosity in Executive Paychecks." *The New York Times*, April 11, p. D1.

———. 1995d. "10 Companies Join in Effort to Lower Bids by HMO's." *The New York Times*, May 23, p. D2.

Fried, Charles. 1969. *An Anatomy of Values*. Cambridge, MA.; Harvard University Press.

Fried, Stephen. 1995. "The Incredible Shrinking Institute." *Philadelphia* 86(April): 67–71, 99–110.

Friedman, M. 1962. *Capitalism and Freedom*. Chicago: University of Chicago Press.

Fritsch, Jane, and Dean Baquet. 1995. "Lack of Oversight Takes Delivery-Room Toll." *The New York Times*, March 6, pp. A1, B4.

Frum, David. 1995. "What To Do About Health Care." *Commentary* 99(June):29–34.

Fry, J., D. W. Light, J. Rodnick, and P. Orton. 1995. *Reviving Primary Care: A US-UK Comparison*. New York: Radcliffe Medical Press.

Fusco, R. 1994. "Home Care: An Emerging Solution to the Healthcare Crisis." *Hospital Topics* 72(Fall):32–36.

Gaylin, W. 1993. "Faulty diagnosis: Why Clinton's Health-Care Plan Won't Cure What Ails Us." *Harper's Magazine*. 287(1721):57–64.

Glaser, W. 1993. "The Competition Vogue and Its Outcomes." *Lancet* 341:805–812.

Goldstein, Amy, and Peter Baker. 1995. "Va. Doctors Forming Their Own HMO; Medical Society Leads Effort to Get More Control over Managed Care." *The Washington Post*, May 4, p. A16.

Gordon, Suzanne. 1995. "Unhealthy Care." *The Nation* 260(May 8):620.

Gorski, Terence T. 1995. "The Evolution of Managed Care." *Treatment Today* 7(Spring): 10–12.

Hadley, J., E. P. Steinberg, and J. Feder. 1991. "Comparison of Uninsured and Privately Insured Hospital Patients: Condition on Admission, Resource Use, and Outcome." *JAMA* 265: 374–9.

Hadorn, D. 1992 *Basic Benefits and Clinical Guidelines*. Boulder CO: Westview Press.

Hammonds, Keith H. 1994. "The New World of Work." *Business Week*, October 17, pp. 76–87.

"Harvard Hospitals to Cut Residents." 1995. *The Press of Atlantic City*, July 17, p. A2.

Health Insurance Association of America, 1995. *Source Book of Health Insurance Data*. Washington, D.C.: HIAA.

Hellander, I., J. Moloo, D. U. Himmelstein, S. Woolhandler, and S. M. Wolfe. 1995. *The Growing Epidemic of Uninsurance*. Chicago: Physicians for a National Health Program.

Henderson, Keith. 1994. "Health-Care Reform Raises Questions of Individual Rights." *The Christian Science Monitor*, March 29, p. 3.

"HHS Proposes Outpatient Prospective Payment." 1995. *Reimbursement Advisor* 10(May): 1.

Hilzenrath, David S. 1994a. "In Corporate Hands, Health Bureaucracy Blooms." *The Washington Post*, September 20, pp. A1, 18.

————. 1994b. "In MD., a Doctor Battles Managed Care Red Tape." *The Washington Post*, September 20, p. 18.

Holahan, J., C. Winterbottom, and S. Rojan. 1995. *The Changing Composition of Health Insurance Coverage in the United States*. Washington, D.C.: The Urban Institute.

"How Managed Care Is Restructuring the Health Care Industry." 1995. A FSCME Department of Public Policy, April.

Hudson, Terese. 1995. "Medicaid: Will the Public Program Neglect the Poor to Pay for the Elderly?" *Hospitals & Health Networks* 69(May 20):28–34.

Iglehart, J. 1976. "The Rising Costs of Health Care: Something Must Be Done, but What?" *National Journal* 8:1458–65.

Iglehart, John K. 1992. "The American Health Care System—Private Insurance." *New England Journal of Medicine* 326:1715–20.

Iglehart, John K. 1995a. "Rapid Changes for Academic Medical Centers." *New England Journal of Medicine* 332:407–11.

Iglehart, J. K. 1995b. "Republicans and the New Politics of Health Care." *New England Journal of Medicine* 332:972–5.

Institute of Medicine. 1988. *The Future of Public Health*. Washington, D.C.: National Academy Press.

Jacobs, Charles. 1995. "7 Hospitals Join, Woo HMOs." *The New York Times*, March 26, pp. 1,10.

Jones, Clarisse. 1995. "Lives in the Balance: Budget Cuts Proposed by Pataki Would Affect Thousands." *The New York Times*, February 5, p. 37.

Judis, J. B. 1995. "Abandoned Surgery: Business and the Failure of Health Care Reform." *American Prospect* 21(spring):65–73.

Kent, Christina. 1995. "Market Forces Cutting Costs; Long Term Effects Unknown." *Medicine & Health Perspectives*, April 17, pp. 1–4.

Kolbert, E. 1995. "Special Interests' Special Weapon: A Seeming Grass-Roots Drive is Quite Often Something Else." *The New York Times*, March 26, 20.

Kongstvedt, Peter. R. 1995. *Essentials of Managed Care*. Gaithersburg, MD.: Aspen Publishers.

Lanzalotti, John A. 1995. "A Way Out of the Current Health Care Dilemma." *Asbury Park Press*, April 13, p. A15.

Lashof, Joyce C. 1994. "Health Care Reform: A Public Health Perspective," In Pauline Vaillancourt Rosenau, ed. *Health Care Reform in the Nineties*. Thousand Oaks, CA: Sage Publications, pp. 69–73.

Levy, Doug. 1995. "Drug Prices Up, but How Much?" *USA Today*, March 16, p. D1.

Lewis, Pearl L. 1995. "Let's Not Push the Old Folks Yet." *The Baltimore Sun*, May 14, p. 4F.

Light, Donald W. 1986. "Corporate Medicine for Profit." *Scientific American* 225:38–45.

———. 1991a. "Effectiveness and Efficiency Under Competition: The Cochrane Test." *British Medical Journal* 303:1253–4.

———. 1991b. "Embedded Inefficiences in Health Care." *Lancet* 338:102–4.

———. 1992a. "The Ethics of Corporate Health Insurance." *Business and Professional Ethics Journal* 10(2):49–62.

———. 1992b. "The Practice and Ethics of Risk-Rated Health Insuranance." *JAMA* 267:2503–8.

———. l993a. "Escaping the Traps of Post-War Western Medicine." *European Journal of Public Health* 3:223–31.

———. 1993b. "US Health Reforms: Cliches, Cost, and Mrs. C." *Lancet* 341(March 27):791.

———. 1994a. "Excluding More and Covering Less: The Health Insurance Industry in the United States." In Nancy F. McKenzie, ed., *Beyond Crisis: Confronting Health Care in the United States.* New York: Penguin Books, pp. 310–20.

———. 1994b. "Health Care Systems and Their Financing." In, J. Walton, J. A. Barondess, and S. Lock, eds., *The New Oxford Medical Companion.* London: Oxford University Press, pp. 355–64.

———. 1994c. "Life, Death and the Insurance Companies." *New England Journal of Medicine* 330:498–500.

———. 1994d. "Managed Care: False and Real Solutions." *Lancet* 344:1197–99.

———. 1994e. "Medical Prices Outrun the Rate of Inflation." *The New York Times*, February 18, p. A26.

Lisa, Joseph P. 1994. *The Assault on Medical Freedom.* Norfolk, Va.: Hampton Roads Publishing Company.

Lueck, Thomas J. 1995. "Giuliani Fiscal Plan Puts Health Care Jobs At Risk." *The New York Times*, February 18, p. A1.

Lurie, Nicole, Ira S. Moscovice, Michael Finch, Jon B. Christianson, and Michael K. Popkin. 1992. "Does Capitation Affect the Health of the Chronically Mentally Ill?" *JAMA* 267:3300.

Mann, Joyce, et al. 1994. *Uncompensated Care: Hospital Responses to Increased Price Competition and Payment Reform.* Santa Monica, Calif.: Rand Corporation.

Marmor, T. R. 1994. *Understanding Health Care Reform.* New Haven, Conn.: Yale University Press.

Maynard, Roberta. 1995. "The Power of Pooling." *Nation's Business*, March, pp. 16–22.

McGregor, A. 1993. "Green Light for Swiss National Health Insurance." *Lancet* 342:857.

McKenna, M. A. J. 1995. "Alternative Medicine: Mainstream Doctors are Now Listening." *Union-News*, June 30, p. C1,2.

Meade, T. W. et al. 1990. "Low Back Pain of Mechanical Origin: Randomised Comparison of Chiropractic and Hospital Outpatient Treatment." *British Medical Journal* 300:1431–7.

Medicaid: States Turn to Managed Care to Improve Access and Control Costs. 1993. Washington, D.C.: U.S. General Accounting Office, March.

Merline, John. 1995. "Reining in Medicare Costs: Pay or Pay." *National Review*, May 29, pp. 45–48.

Meyer, Harris. 1994. "HMOs May Improve Preventive Care, but Reform Must Create Proper Incentives." *American Medical News* 37(May 23):3

Milhiser, Ellen Altman. 1995. "Congressional Budget Debate on Medicare Heats Up." *Reimbursement Advisor* 10(June): 1–4.

Myers, Steven Lee. 1995. "Rating Agency Issues Warning on City Hospitals Corporations." *The New York Times*, February 18, p. A4.

Neus, Elizabeth. 1995. "Turnovers in HMOs Spark Debate over Doctor Coverage." *Courier-Post*, February 6, p. 3B.

Nixon, J. Peter. 1994. "Health Care Reform: A Labor Perspective" In Rosenau, P.V. (ed.) *Health Care Reform in the Nineties*. Thousand Oaks, CA: Sage Publications, pp. 202–12.

Nordgren, Robert A. 1995. "The Case Against Managed Care and for a Single-Payer System." *JAMA* 273:79.

Nozick, R. 1974. *Anarchy, State, and Utopia*. New York: Basic Books.

"Nurses Protest Layoffs, Care Cut." 1995. *The Atlantic City Press*, April 1, p. A2.

Offner, Paul. 1994. "Willing and Able." *The New Republic*, November 14, pp. 11–12.

Olmos, David R. 1995. "Shift to HMOs Brings Warnings on Abuses." *Philadelphia Inquirer*, March 22, p. 1.

Osher, F. C., and J. B. Christianson. 1994. "Health Maintenance Organizations, Health Care Reform, and the Persons with Serious Mental Illness." *Hospital Community Psychiatry* 45(September):898–905.

Pallararito, Karen. 1994. "Covering the Risks of Capitation." *Modern Healthcare* May 16, p. 44.

Patrick, Donald L. and Pennifer Erickson. 1993. *Health Status and Health Policy*. New York: Oxford University Prress.

Patterson, Mary Jo. 1995. "Mental-Health Experts Debate Managed Care." *The Star Ledger*, March 5, p. 51.

Payer, L. 1988. *Medicine and Culture*. New York: Penguin.

———. 1992. *Disease-Mongers*. New York: Wiley.

Pear, R. 1994. "States Again Try Health Changes as Congress Fails." *The New York Times*, September 16, p. A1.

Pearsall, Richard. 1995. "Physicians Fight Loss of Control to Businesses." *Courier-Post*, April 16, p. 3E.

Perednia, D. A. 1995. "Telemedicine Technology and Clinical Applications" *JAMA* 273:483–8.

Peters, W. P., and M.C. Rogers. 1994. "Variation in Approval by Insurance Companies of Coverage for Autologous Bone Marrow Transplantation for Breast Cancer." *New England Journal of Medicine* 330:473–8.

Peterson, Iver. 1994. "Health Care and Hospital Chains; Small Institutions Choose Survival over Independence." *The New York Times*, November 15, p. B1.

"Physician Corp. of America to Buy Health Plus Inc." 1994. *The New York Times*, November 22, p. C5, D5.

Priester, R. 1992. "A Values Framework for Health System Reform." *Health Affairs* 11, no. 1:84–107.

"Prognosis Not Clear on Affect of Nurse Cuts." 1995. *The Atlantic City Press*, July 30, p. A6.

"Public Health Threatened" 1995. *The Nation's Health* 25(March):S1.

Quinn, Jane Bryan. 1994. "Health Care Report Cards." *Newsweek*, October 17, p. 57.

Quint, Michael. 1995. "Health Plans Force Changes in the Way Doctors Are Paid." *The New York Times*, February 9, p. A1.

Rasell, M. E. 1995. "Cost Sharing in Health Insurance—a reexamination." *New England Journal of Medicine* 332:1164–1168.

Rawls, J. 1971. *A Theory of Justice*. Cambridge, MA: Harvard University Press.

———. 1993. *Political Liberalism*. New York: Columbia Unversity Press.

Reinhardt, Uwe E. 1984 "Are Americans Really as Mean as They Seem? pp. 7–30 In *Uncompensated Care in a Competitive Environment: Whose Problem is it?* Washington, DC: Department of Health and Human Services, National Council on Health Planning and Development (HRP-0906304)

———. 1993. "Reorganizing the Financial Flows in American Health Care." *Health Affairs* 12(supp.):172–193.

———. 1995a. "Turning Our Gaze From Bread and Circus Games." *Health Affairs* 14(Spring):33–36.

———. 1995b. "When Trenton Plays Obstetrician." *The New York Times*, July 9, p. 15.

Rice, T., E. R. Brown, and R. Wyn, 1993. "Holes in the Jackson Hole Approach to Health Care Reform." *JAMA* 270:1357–62.

Rivlin, A. 1974. "Agreed: Here Comes National Health Insurance." *The New York Times Magazine*. (July 21): pp.8, 35, 46–50, 54.

RWJ (The Robert Wood Johnson Foundation). 1995. "Sick People in Managed Care Have Difficulty Getting Services and Treatment, New Survey Reports" News frrom the Robert Wood Johnson Foundation. Princeton, NJ: RWJ Foundation.

Roberts, Marc J. 1993. *Your Money or Your Life: The Health Care Crisis Explained.* New York: Doubleday.

Rosenbaum, David E. 1995. "In the War of Politics, Medicare Spending Has Become the Latest Battlefield." *The New York Times*, May 2, p. A14.

Rosenthal, Elisabeth. 1995. "Young Doctors Find Specialist Jobs Hard to Find." *The New York Times*, April 15, p. 1.

Rothman, D. J. 1993. "A Century of Failure: Health Care Reform in America." *Journal of Health Politics, Policy, and Law* 18, no. 2:271–86.

Russell, L. 1986. *Is Prevention Better than Cure?* Washington, D.C.: Brookings Institution.

———. 1994. *Educated Guesses: Making Policy About Medical Screening Tests.* Berkeley: University of California Press and The Milbank Memorial Fund.

Russell, Suzanne C. 1995. "Bone Marrow Treatment Coverage Bill Gains." *The News Tribune*, February 7, p. A9.

Sabin, J. E., and N. Daniels. 1994. "Determining 'Medical Necessity' in Mental Health Practice." *Hastings Center Report* 24, no. 6:5–13.

Sack, Kevin. 1995. "Public Hospitals around Country Cut Basic Service." *The New York Times*, August 20, pp. A1,24.

"Scherer's Pact with Marquest." 1993. *The Wall Street Journal*, March 18, p. C17.

Schlesinger, M., and Tae-ku Lee, 1993. "Is Health Care Different? Popular Support for Federal Health and Social Policies." *Journal of Health Politics, Policy, and Law* 18, no. 3:551–628.

Schroeder, Steven A., 1994. "The Presidents' Message: Cost Containment." *Annual Report For 1994 of the Robert Wood Johnson Foundation*. Princeton, N.J.: RWJ Foundation.

Schwartz, Matthew. 1995. "Medicare Encouraging HMOs to Enroll the Elderly." *National Underwriter Life & Health—Financial Services Edition*, February 6, p. 3.

Sen, A. 1990. "Justice: Means vs Freedom." *Philosophy and Public Affairs* 19:111–21.
———. 1992. *Inequality Reexamined*. Cambridge, MA: Harvard University Press.
Somerville, Janice. 1994. "Doctors Treating the Poor Hit Hard by Kentucky Cuts." *American Medical News*, December 12, p. 3.
Starfield, B. 1993. *Primary Care: Concept, Evaluation, and Policy*. New York: Oxford University Press.
Starr, Paul. 1982. *The Social Transformation of American Medicine*. New York: Basic Books.
———. 1995. "What Happened to Health Care Reform?" *American Prospect* 20:20–31.
Stayn, Susan J. 1994. "Securing Access to Care on Health Maintenance Organizations: Toward a Uniform Model of Grievance and Appeal Procedures" *Columbia Law Review* 94(June):1674–720.
Stewart, Angela. 1995. "Three Hospitals to Combine for Biggest Network." *The Star Ledger*, May 5, p. 1,16.
Stoddard, J. J., R. F. Peter, and P. W. Newacheck. 1994. "Health Insurance Status and Ambulatory Care for Children." *New England Journal of Medicine* 330:1321–25.
Stone, D. A. 1993. "The Struggle for the Soul of Health Insurance." *Journal of Health Politics, Policy, and Law* 18:287–318.
Stovall, Ellen, John F. Hughes, and Martin W. Schwartz. 1994. "Choice and Health Insurance." *The Washington Post*, April 18, p. A18.
"Study Before Joining 'Managed Care' " *The Washington Post* 1995 (May 7).
Sugg, Diana. 1995. "HMO Marketeers' Medicaid Tactics Probed by State." *The Baltimore Sun*, May 14, p. 1, 21.
Sullivan, Joseph F. 1994. "New Jersey Plans to Cut Payments for Medicaid 20%." *The New York Times*, November 23, p. 1.
Toner, Robin. 1995. "GOP Moves Health Debate to Medicare." *The New York Times*, February 12, p. 1.
Toner, Robin, and Robert Pear. 1995. "Medicare, Turning 30, Won't Be What It Was." *The New York Times*, July 23, p. 1, 24.
Tumulty, Karen. 1994. "Push for Cost Controls on Health Takes a Back Seat." *Los Angeles Times*, August 11, p. A1.
U.S. Government Accounting Office. 1993. *Managed Health Care: Effects on Employers' Costs Difficult to Measure*. Washington, D.C.: GAO.
Valdez-Dapena, Peter. 1995. "Doctors with Union Cards." *Business Week*, January 23, p. 101.
Watson, Tom. 1995. "Budget Troubles Threaten Health of Public Hospitals." *USA Today*, March 29, p. 1.
Weiner, Joshua M. 1994. "The American Health Care System in the Year 2000." Unpublished paper. Washington, D.C.: The Brookings Institution.
Weinstein, Michael M. 1994. "The Freedom to Choose Doctors: What Freedom?" *The New York Times Magazine*, March 27, pp. 64–5.
Weissman, Joel S., and Arnold M. Epstein. 1994. *Falling through the Safety Net: Insurance Status and Access to Health Care*. Baltimore, Md.: Johns Hopkins University Press.
White, Jane H. 1994 "Health System Changes in the Absence of National Reform." *Health Progress* 75(December):10.
White House Domestic Policy Council. 1993. *The President's Health Security Plan*. New York: Times Books.

Whitlow, Joan. 1995. "Doctors' Practices Going to the Highest Bidder." *The Star Ledger*, February 12, pp. 1,12.

Wikler, Daniel. 1978. "Persuasion and Coercion for Health: Issue in Government Efforts to Change Life Style" *Milbank Memorial Fund Quarterly: Health and Society* 56: 303–38.

Winslow, Ron. 1993. "Managed Care Spells Suspicion, Confusion for Some Consumers; Minneapolis Group Interviews Uncover Distrust of the Role Played by Financial Motives," *The Wall Street Journal*, Mat24, B6.

Winslow, Ron. 1994. "Health-Care Report Cards Are Getting Low Grades from Some Focus Groups." *The Wall Street Journal*, May 19, p. B1.

———. 1995a. "Medical Upheaval; Welfare Recipients Are a Hot Commodity in Managed Care Now." *The Wall Street Journal*, April 12, p. A1.

———. 1995b. "New 'Report Card' on Health Plans Uses Standardized Criteria, Audited Data." *The Wall Street Journal*, February 24, p. B6.

Wofford, H. 1994. "Cooper Pooper." *New Republic*, February 7, pp. 19–20.

World Bank. 1993. *Investing in Health: World Development Report 1993*. Washington, D.C.: The World Bank.

World Health Organization (WHO). 1946. Preamble to Constitution of WHO. *Official Record of World Health Organization* 2:100.

Wysong, J. A., and T. Abel. 1990. "Universal Health Insurance and High-Risk Groups in West Germany: Implications for U.S. Health Policy." *Milbank Quarterly* 68:527–60.

Yarborough, Mary H. 1995. "It's a Matter of Crime and Cost." *HR Focus* 72, no. 3:9–10.

Index

and universal access (minimizing
nonfinancial barriers), 40
formal vs. fair, 19–20, 22. *See also* Fair
equality of opportunity
and health care, 21–23, 25, 27, 29, 32–33
vs. individual traits as benefit, 47
and Libertarian viewpoint, 30
and Rawls' veil of ignorance, 29–30
and tiering, 27
Equitable financing—by ability to pay
(benchmark), 32–33, 50–53, 68
current trends scored on, 150, 164
insurance reforms scored on, 92–96, 97,
132
Equitable financing—community-rated
contributions (benchmark), 32–33,
44–50, 68
current trends scored on, 149–50, 164
insurance reforms scored on, 88–92, 97,
131
Erickson, Pennifer, 26
Ethics Working Group of Health Care Task
Force, 30, 171
Evaluation, public procedures for, 117–18,
158–59
Evans, R. G., 15–16, 88
Expenditures for health care. *See* cost,
health care

Fair equality of opportunity, 19–20, 22, 31.
See also Equality of opportunity
and equitable financing, 45
and progressive taxation, 33
and solidarity principle, 46
Fairness, 3, 9, 12–13, 31.
and affordability or feasibility, 87
and American health care system, 134, 167
and American values, 15, 18, 20–21
and burdens, 44
and Clinton/103rd Congress health care
debate, 8–9
deliberations about submerged, 11–12
and economic efficiency, 11–12
and empirical assumptions, 31, 36, 53
and empirical vs. moral beliefs, 31, 36
and employer mandate, 9–10
and equality vs. efficiency or liberty,
23–24
equality of opportunity as, 19–20. *See also*
Equality of opportunity
and financing, 10–11
and public debate, 34
Rawls' theory of justice-as, 51
social vs. actuarial, 46
and universal access, 35–36
and wasted resources, 53, 56

Feder, J., 8, 38, 48
Federal Trade Commission, 160–61
Fein, Esther B., 145, 148
Feingold, E., 104
Feldstein, P. J., 15
Felsenthal, E., 160
Financial efficiency. *See* Value for money—
financial efficiency
Financing, and fairness, 10–11
Findlay, Steven, 156
Fisher, F. C., 147
Fisher, Ian, 145, 148
Fisher, Mary Jane, 141
Flat tax, 32, 52
Flood, A. B., 63
Foreign nations, health care systems of, 74
Britain, 27–28, 56, 61, 80, 82, 102–03
Canada, 27, 56, 73
Germany, 43–44, 61, 90, 112
Holland, 112
Japan, 61, 112
Norway, 27
Formal equality of opportunity, 19
For-profit health care organizations, 55–56,
140, 158, 168
Fowler, F. J., Jr., 42
Frank, Richard G., 147
Franks, P., 8, 38, 48
Fraud and abuse, 100
and current trends, 157–58
need to reduce, 57
and reform proposals, 114–16
Free-loading, 36
Free market. *See* Market-based approach
Freudenheim, Milt, 8, 143, 145, 154–155
Fried, Charles, 25
Fried, Stephen, 142, 152
Friedman, Milton, 12
Fritsch, Jane, 153
Fry, J., 103
"Function," meaning of, 26
Fusco, R., 142
Future of U.S. health care, 167–73

German health care system
and community rating, 90
global budgets in, 112
level of expenditures in, 61
and supplemental insurance, 43–44
Glaser, W., 11
Global health care budget, 60–62
lack of, 39
in McDermott/Wellstone bill, 73, 111–12,
122
and public attitude, 171
Gold, M. R., 8, 38, 48